Certified Medical Administrative Assistant (CMAA) Study Guide

EDITION 2.0

AUTHOR
Marilyn Fenichel

REVIEWER
Lisa K. Smith, CMA, RMA

COPY EDITOR
Kelly Von Lunen

GRAPHIC DESIGNERS
Spring Lenox
Randi Janell Hardy

ADDITIONAL CONTRIBUTORS
Derek Prater
Kaitlyn Mackey
Brant Stacey
Morgan Smith
Nicole Lobdell

IMPORTANT NOTICE TO THE READER

Assessment Technologies Institute, LLC, is the publisher of this publication. The content of this publication is for informational and educational purposes only and may be modified or updated by the publisher at any time. This publication is not providing medical advice and is not intended to be a substitute for professional medical advice, diagnosis, or treatment. The publisher has designed this publication to provide accurate information regarding the subject matter covered; however, the publisher is not responsible for errors, omissions, or for any outcomes related to the use of the contents of this book and makes no guarantee and assumes no responsibility or liability for the use of the products and procedures described or the correctness, sufficiency, or completeness of stated information, opinions, or recommendations. The publisher does not recommend or endorse any specific tests, providers, products, procedures, processes, opinions, or other information that may be mentioned in this publication. Treatments and side effects described in this book may not be applicable to all people; likewise, some people may require a dose or experience a side effect that is not described herein. Drugs and medical devices are discussed that may have limited availability controlled by the Food and Drug Administration (FDA) for use only in a research study or clinical trial. Research, clinical practice, and government regulations often change the accepted standard in this field. When consideration is being given to use of any drug in the clinical setting, the health care provider or reader is responsible for determining FDA status of the drug, reading the package insert, and reviewing prescribing information for the most up-to-date recommendations on dose, precautions, and contraindications and determining the appropriate usage for the product. Any references in this book to procedures to be employed when rendering emergency care to the sick and injured are provided solely as a general guide. Other or additional safety measures may be required under particular circumstances. This book is not intended as a statement of the standards of care required in any particular situation, because circumstances and a patient's physical condition can vary widely from one emergency to another. Nor is it intended that this book shall in any way advise personnel concerning legal authority to perform the activities or procedures discussed. Such specific determination should be made only with the aid of legal counsel. Some images in this book feature models. These models do not necessarily endorse, represent, or participate in the activities represented in the images. THE PUBLISHER MAKES NO REPRESENTATIONS OR WARRANTIES OF ANY KIND, WHETHER EXPRESS OR IMPLIED, WITH RESPECT TO THE CONTENT HEREIN. THIS PUBLICATION IS PROVIDED AS-IS, AND THE PUBLISHER AND ITS AFFILIATES SHALL NOT BE LIABLE FOR ANY ACTUAL, INCIDENTAL, SPECIAL, CONSEQUENTIAL, PUNITIVE, OR EXEMPLARY DAMAGES RESULTING, IN WHOLE OR IN PART, FROM THE READER'S USE OF, OR RELIANCE UPON, SUCH CONTENT.

INTRODUCTION

About $3.8 trillion was spent on health care in the U.S. in 2014. Health care is big business. Qualified medical administrative assistants, like you, will continue to be in demand. Health care practitioners rely on skilled administrative staff for the financial health of their business. Medical administrative assistants qualify for employment in a variety of settings, including hospitals, clinics, insurance companies, dental offices, and private provider offices, as well as county and government offices. Accepting the challenge to become a part of this growing field requires dedication and a willingness to continually update your skills. Possessing a medical administrative assistant certification will help you support a successful career in this field. This study guide will help you prepare for the National Healthcare Association (NHA) Certified Medical Administrative Assistant (CMAA) certification examination.

In order to sit for the CMAA examination, you must have a high school diploma or a GED and complete a training program. However, you may substitute 1 year of medical administrative assistant experience in lieu of attending a formal training program. With this option, you must provide documentation that you worked as a medical administrative assistant for at least 1 year. If you meet these criteria, you may register for the examination online at http://www.nhanow.com/medical-admin-assistant.aspx.

The CMAA exam consists of 110 scored multiple-choice questions and 20 unscored pretest questions. If your school is a registered NHA test site, you may be able to take a proctored exam via computer or in paper-pencil format. You also have the option to take the exam via computer at a PSI testing center. For more information about exam eligibility, refer to the Candidate Handbook in the Certifications section of www.nhanow.com. The key instructional content, or body of each chapter, follows the CMAA test plan. Following the key instructional content, there is a chapter summary that recaps the main points within the chapter and drill questions that assess your knowledge of the chapter subjects. A terms and definitions section at the end of this handbook defines the key words highlighted throughout.

NHA Certified Medical Administrative Assistant (CMAA) Detailed Test Plan based on the 2014 Job Analysis Study

The tasks under each content domain are examples that are representative of the content. Items reflective of these stated tasks may or may not appear on the examination. Additionally, items that are reflective of tasks other than those included in the above outline may appear on the examination, as long as they represent information that is considered part of the major content domain by experts in the medical administrative assistant profession.

1. Scheduling   Scored Items: 19

A. Evaluate different types of patient scheduling
- Identify the patient (e.g., the same last name, same first AND last name, same date of birth).
- Interpret the purpose of the visit.
- Arrange the procedures in the scheduling book.
- Knowledge of wave booking
- Knowledge of double-booking
- Knowledge of modified wave
- Knowledge of stream/time-specific
- Knowledge of open booking
- Knowledge of cluster or categorization booking

B. Determine scheduling needs of the facility, as well as new and established patients
- Knowledge of how to input new patient information
- Identify type of service needed by the patient.
- Knowledge of availability on the provider's schedule (e.g., physician and nurse)
- Obtain referrals.
- Knowledge of appointment intervals
- Knowledge of physicians' preferences, needs, and schedule matrix
- Knowledge of block scheduling
- Knowledge of nurses' preferences, needs, and schedule
- Identify dates and times when the schedule needs to be blocked out for the facility.

C. Follow protocol for no-show, missed, cancelled, or follow-up appointments
- Knowledge of fees
- Knowledge of follow-up procedures for no-show, missed, and cancelled appointments
- Knowledge of office policies related to charges for missed appointments
- Check with physician to determine if a patient can be seen.
- Reschedule for later appointments.
- Knowledge of how to document a no-show, missed, or cancelled appointment
- Send out notifications for no-show and missed appointments.

D. Arrange for diagnostic testing and procedures
- Call for pre-authorization for testing and procedures.
- Check for referrals prior to appointment.
- Knowledge of participating or non-participating facilities to arrange for diagnostic testing and procedures

- Verify patient billing address for scheduling needs.
- Verify best method of contact for scheduling appointments.
- Provide patient with instructions for pre-testing or diagnostic procedures.
- Schedule pre-admission testing.
- Ensure patient has the correct address of the facility.
- Ensure patient has the correct name of the referred physician.
- Document information in patient chart.
- Follow-up with patient to ensure compliance with physician's instructions.

E. Confirm future appointments
- Follow HIPAA guidelines (e.g., what should or should not be disclosed when scheduling and confirming future appointments).
- Instruct patient to bring insurance and identification to the appointment.
- Verify patient's insurance is participating with physician's office.
- Knowledge of how to document a no-show, missed, or cancelled appointment
- Check for referrals prior to appointment.
- Inform patient of copay requirement.

2. Patient Intake   Scored Items: 18

A. Confirm demographic information with patient
- Maintain appropriate demographic data (e.g., address, phone number, date of birth, insurance information).
- Check that the patient's Protected Health Information (PHI) has been entered.
- Confirm the patient's advanced directives.
- Knowledge of special needs in regards to special paperwork (e.g., visually impaired patients, language barrier patients)
- Ensure demographic form is signed.
- Knowledge of best method of contact for confirming demographic information

B. Verify insurance information
- Verify coverage benefits.
- Verify copay.
- Review insurance card.
- Review form of photo identification.
- Verify changes in coverage.
- Verify whether patient has secondary and/or tertiary coverage.
- Knowledge of the birthday rule
- Verify policyholder.
- Determine which laboratory is the appropriate facility for a patient to use.
- Determine benefit information.
- Identify the difference between the guarantor and the patient, if it exists.
- Knowledge of basic coding (e.g., ICD, CPT)
- Ability to communicate with insurance company

C. Ensure forms are updated or completed
- Ensure forms are signed (e.g., assignment of benefits, advanced directives, living will, health history, consent to release information, records release, HIPAA release, financial responsibility, DNR, health care surrogate).

D. Prepare encounter form
- Knowledge of other practitioners and physicians for referrals
- Basic knowledge of procedures performed in the back office
- Verify information on encounter form.
- Recognize, but do not interpret, basic coding (e.g., ICD, CPT).

E. Prepare daily charts
- Retrieve and file the record.
- Create medical record.
- Knowledge of how to retrieve future appointment schedules
- Ensure delivery to the proper physician.
- Match the correct patient to the correct chart.
- Update the patient's chart with progress notes.

3. Office Logistics
Scored Items: 12

A. File medical records
- Knowledge of filing systems (e.g., electronic, alphabetical procedures, terminal digit procedures [such as primary, secondary, and tertiary])
- Ability to cross-reference charts
- Basic knowledge of scanning documents
- Basic knowledge of correlation of charts (e.g., labs categorized under laboratories, prescriptions categorized under Prescriptions)
- Basic knowledge of EHR/EMR (Electronic Health Records/Electronic Medical Records)

B. Perform financial procedures
- Collect copayments.
- Create statements (e.g., office visit invoices, pre-invoices).
- Create receipt for payment.
- Knowledge of basic financial terminology (e.g., copay, deductibles, co-insurance, fee schedule)
- Use of petty cash
- Basic knowledge of bookkeeping system (e.g., double or single entry)
- Complete day sheet

C. Evaluate mail deliveries
- Sort and distribute mail.
- Knowledge of different classes of mail (e.g., registered, certified, first-class, priority, FedEx, USPS)
- Verify contents of package against package slip.

4. Compliance
Scored Items: 16

A. Follow HIPAA guidelines
- Ensure patient's privacy and security of protected health information.
- Ensure charts are properly secured (e.g., displayed with personal information covered).
- Use a HIPAA-compliant sign-in sheet.
- Knowledge of what information is not private for authorities and health departments (e.g., child abuse, STDs/STIs, gunshot wounds, HIV)
- Knowledge of record release forms
- Knowledge of who can access patient's chart
- Proper use of passwords
- Knowledge of peer-to-peer information
- Follow HIPAA guidelines for covered and non-covered entities.
- Knowledge of appropriate discussion of medical information (e.g., when and where)
- Knowledge of proper verification of medical information (e.g., what to release and what not to release when verifying information)
- Knowledge of penalties for violating HIPAA practices
- Document release of information (e.g., when and to whom information can be released)
- Knowledge of PHI standards

B. Follow OSHA guidelines
- Adhere to OSHA guidelines.
- Knowledge of MSDS
- Knowledge of how to report an OSHA incident
- Knowledge of the evacuation plans and emergency procedures

C. Follow the Center for Medicare/Medicaid Services (CMS) guidelines
- Report Medicare/Medicaid fraud
- Awareness of consequences of fraud
- Knowledge of the difference between Medicare and Medicaid
- Recognize the CMS-1500 form
- Recognize the UB-04

5. Patient Education
Scored Items: 11

A. Explain the Patients' Bill of Rights
- Explain to patient that medical decisions are made by physicians.
- Explain to patient that he/she has the right to go to a medical specialist.
- Explain to patient that he/she has the right to keep the same physician through a procedure or treatment.
- Knowledge of who owns the medical record
- Knowledge of disability practices (e.g., ADA compliance)
- Compare and contrast different forms of consent (e.g., implied consent, verbal consent, written consent, expressed consent, implied minor consent).
- Knowledge of basic medical law and ethics (e.g., assault and battery, patient abandonment)
- Explain to a patient that he/she has the right to be seen by another physician

B. Explain the patients' insurance responsibilities
- Explain the difference between copayments and coinsurance.
- Explain deductibles.
- Explain allowed amounts.
- Basic knowledge of insurance practices
- Explain the difference between federal and private insurance.
- Explain an Advanced Beneficiary Notice (ABN)
- Knowledge of the contents of an Explanation of Benefits (EOB)

C. Explain pre- and post-instructions for testing and procedures
- Provide written documentation on procedure
- Reiterate to the patient the physician's instructions

6. General Office Policies and Procedures   Scored Items: 15

A. Perform office opening and closing procedures
- Check internal and external messages (e.g., phones, emails, faxes).
- Check that charts are prepared and ready for the day (or next day).
- Check that the amount of petty cash for the day is correct.
- Direct and redirect phones to and from answering service to office.
- Ensure day sheets are balanced.
- Ensure equipment is turned on at open and off at close.
- Clean up reception area.
- Back up data.
- Order supplies.

B. Greet patients upon arrival
- Greet patients with a positive attitude.
- Identify type of visit (e.g., sick or well).
- Identify type of patient (i.e., new or existing).
- Ensure front office is free of obstacles.
- Acknowledge patients upon arrival.
- Notify patients of wait time.

C. Apply telephone etiquette
- Introduce facility and self.
- Identify type of caller.
- Identify caller's need.
- Check on callers with extended hold times.

D. Create correspondences
- Knowledge of templates
- Knowledge of word processing
- Knowledge of different types of letters
- Knowledge of different types of correspondences
- Create letters.
- Use proper greetings and salutations.
- Apply proper postage.
- Obtain required signatures (e.g., who should sign the correspondence?).

E. Demonstrate basic computer skills
- Knowledge of e-mail system (e.g., Microsoft Outlook)
- Knowledge of word processing (e.g., Microsoft Word)
- Knowledge of spreadsheets (e.g., Microsoft Excel)
- Knowledge of internet (e.g., social media, web searching)
- Use of hardware (e.g., copiers, fax machines, scanners)
- Basic HIPAA regulations for the use of the computer
- Skills at computer software

7. Basic Medical Terminology   Scored Items: 19

A. Use medical terminology to communicate with patients and physicians.
- Basic knowledge of pronunciation
- Basic knowledge of spelling
- Basic knowledge of the meaning of terms

B. Recognize abbreviations and acronyms used to complete administrative duties
- Identify the meaning of abbreviations and acronyms (e.g., HX, Pt, H&P, Dx, SOAP, HIPAA, CC, Rx, PHI, CDC, AMA, HMO, PPO).
- Use of abbreviations and acronyms to complete basic administrative duties

C. Use word parts (i.e., prefixes, roots, suffixes) to define medical terminology
- Basic knowledge of prefixes (e.g., a-, an-, pre-, post-, hyper-, hypo-, peri-, endo-, exo-)
- Basic knowledge of roots (e.g., cardi/o, vascul/o, gastr/o, nephr/o, hepat/o)
- Basic knowledge of suffixes (e.g., -logy, -itis, -osis, -pathy, -ist, -graph)

Table of Contents

CHAPTER 5
Patient Education — 73

CHAPTER 1
Scheduling

OVERVIEW

The medical administrative assistant field is broad and versatile. Professionals are trained to perform a wide range of administrative tasks. Medical administrative assistants greet patients and obtain basic information, enter the information into the patient's medical record, answer the telephone, schedule appointments, update medical records, and handle all types of correspondence. They also must be familiar with regulations established by the Health Insurance Portability and Accountability Act (HIPAA), the U.S. Occupational Safety and Health Administration (OSHA), and the Clinical Laboratory Improvement Act (CLIA), as well as the requirements of insurance plans. Finally, medical administrative assistants need to have an understanding of basic medical terminology.

This chapter focuses on one part of the job's administrative side: scheduling appointments. This topic includes different kinds of scheduling; determining the scheduling needs of providers, patients, and the facility; arranging for diagnostic testing and procedures; and confirming future appointments.

By the end of this chapter, you should be able to answer the following questions.

1. What are three advantages of computer scheduling?
2. When are patients scheduled in wave booking?
3. How are patients scheduled in cluster or categorization booking?
4. When scheduling appointments, what factors need to be taken into account?
5. An office schedules appointments every 20 minutes, with 30 minutes blocked off for lunch. However, the provider usually spends 30 minutes with each patient and takes 20 minutes for lunch. The waiting room is usually full. How could this office run more smoothly?
6. True or False: Medical practices never charge for no-shows.
7. Why is automated call routing a good strategy for preventing no-shows?
8. A patient was scheduled for an appointment, but the doctor was called away due to an emergency. How should the medical administrative assistant handle the situation?
9. Why is it important to document no-shows?
10. Why is it important to get preauthorization if the patient's insurance requires you to do so?

TYPES OF PATIENT SCHEDULING

Scheduling is an important variable in ensuring that a medical practice functions well. The challenge is matching the patients' needs with the provider's preferences and habits, the amount of space available at each facility the practice uses, and the duration of the office visits. For example, if appointments are being scheduled 15 minutes apart but the provider is typically spending 20 to 25 minutes with each patient, then the schedule must be adjusted.

Before scheduling a procedure, the medical administrative assistant must make sure that the provider, the equipment needed, and a room are available. The administrative assistant also must know how long the procedure will take. This information is important because the provider's reimbursement from insurance companies is partly based on the amount of time the patient is required to stay in the office.

Computer Scheduling

In many practices, computer scheduling has replaced the hard-copy appointment book. Some computer systems display only available and scheduled times, while others show length and type of appointment required and day or time preferences. With those programs, the program can select the best appointment time based on the information in the computer. For this reason, it is important that the patient's first and last name and birth date are entered correctly into the system. Without complete patient information, the medical administrative assistant might not be able to select the proper appointment type or providers. It is also essential to crosscheck names and birthdays to look for patients with overlapping information.

The computer also can track future appointments that have already been scheduled. For example, if a patient calls to check on an appointment, the system can search by the patient's name to find the time and date. The providers' daily schedule can be printed, including the patients' names, telephone numbers, and reason for the visit. If necessary, multiple copies of the schedules can be printed.

Book Scheduling

Many different kinds of appointment books are available. Some show an entire week at a glance and are color-coded, with a specific color used for each day of the week. This feature can be helpful when scheduling return appointments. For example, if the patient needs to return 2 weeks from Wednesday, the medical administrative assistant can easily find the right day by using the color-coding.

In addition, the appointment books can include multiple columns. These extra columns may be used to track appointments for each doctor in the practice.

Medical administrative assistants should always include the patient's name and phone number in the appointment book. Sometimes providers ask that the reason for the visit be included as well. That might not be necessary, however, if the assistant references the time and duration of the appointment.

The information in appointment books should be written in pencil. This makes it easier to make changes. Because the appointment book may be used for legal purposes, it must be easy to read and accurate.

Types of Booking

Along with determining the format used for scheduling, medical practices need to decide the type of scheduling they want to use. Types include the following.

- Wave booking
- Modified wave booking
- Double-booking
- Stream/time-specific scheduling
- Open booking
- Cluster or categorization booking

An individual practice may rely on one type, or use a mix of types to ensure that the day's "flow" runs smoothly.

The following sections describe each kind of scheduling approach.

Wave Booking

Instead of scheduling individual patients for 20-minute intervals, patients are scheduled at the same time each hour. The purpose of this approach is to create short-term flexibility each hour. The assumption is that the time needed for each patient will average out over the course of the day. Patients are seen in the order of their arrival, which is often tracked by a sign-in sheet. As a result, one person's late arrival doesn't disrupt the schedule for the day.

FIGURE 1.1 *Wave booking example*

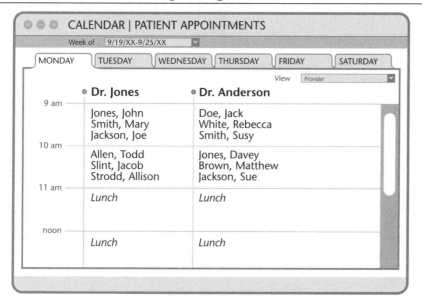

Modified Wave Booking

Wave booking can be modified in a couple of different ways. One example of this approach is to schedule two patients to come at 9 a.m. and one patient at 9:30. This hourly cycle is repeated throughout the day. Another approach is to schedule patients to arrive at given intervals during the first half of the hour and none for the second half of the hour. In this way, the second half of the hour can be used for patients who need extra time.

FIGURE 1.2 *Modified wave booking example*

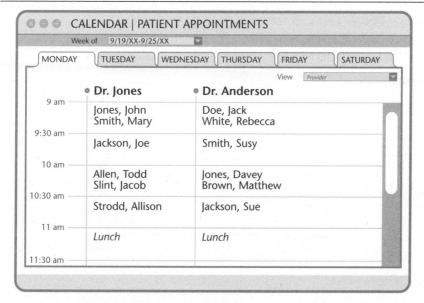

---

wave booking. Patients are scheduled at the same time each hour to create short-term flexibility each hour.

modified wave booking. Wave booking can be modified in a couple of different ways. One example of this approach is to schedule two patients to come at 9 a.m. and one patient at 9:30 a.m. This hourly cycle is repeated throughout the day.

Double-Booking

Double-booking is when two patients are scheduled to come at the same time to see the same provider. This is typically not considered a good approach to scheduling. However, it can be used if both appointments will be only 5 minutes long and a 15-minute interval is reserved for both patients. But if both patients require 15 minutes, a 30-minute interval must be set aside.

If two patients are scheduled to come to the office at the same time but not to see the same provider, this is not considered double-booking. An example of this is when one patient sees the provider and the second receives an allergy shot from a nurse.

double-booking. Two patients are scheduled to come at the same time to see the same physician.

stream/time-specific scheduling. Scheduling patients for specific times at regular intervals. The amount of time allotted depends on the reason for the visit.

open booking (tidal wave scheduling). Patients are not scheduled for a specific time, but told to come in at intermittent times. They are seen in the order in which they arrive.

cluster or categorization booking. Booking a number of patients who have specific needs together at the same time of day.

Stream/Time-Specific Scheduling

This approach involves scheduling patients for specific times at regular intervals. The amount of time allotted depends on the reason for the visit.

Open Booking

Practices that use this approach, also called *tidal wave scheduling*, do not schedule patients for a specific time. Instead, patients are told to come in at intermittent times. Then they will be seen in the order in which they arrive. Some facilities allow online and telephone check-ins so patients can be notified when their turn is coming up.

Providers who use this method say that it eliminates the annoyance of broken appointments and offices not running on schedule. Nonetheless, few practices in large metropolitan cities use this approach. It is more commonly seen in rural areas, laboratories, imaging facilities, and emergency departments.

The problem with this approach is that the waiting room can fill up quickly, resulting in long wait times for patients. Patients also may arrive in waves, causing some parts of the day to be very busy and other parts very slow. The lack of predictable flow can make it difficult for office duties to get done efficiently.

Cluster or Categorization Booking

This approach refers to booking different times of the day for specific kinds of patients. For example, an internal medicine practice may opt to reserve all morning appointments for complete physical examinations and the afternoon for sick patient visits. A surgeon might reserve 1 day each week to seeing only referral patients. Obstetricians may schedule pregnant patients on different days from gynecology patients.

Depending on the nature of the practice, different groupings may work better than others. Trial-and-error experimentation is often the best way to determine the best groupings. When organized properly, this approach can be very attractive to many providers.

What is the difference between wave booking and stream/time-specific scheduling?

ANSWER: Wave booking is when multiple patients are scheduled at the same time and seen on a first-come first-served basis. Stream/time-specific scheduling is when patients are scheduled at a set time, with the amount of time scheduled contingent on the reason for the visit.

DETERMINING SCHEDULING NEEDS

When scheduling appointments, the medical administrative assistant must keep three sets of needs in mind: the patients', providers', and facility's. Patients have different reasons for visiting the doctor, and some visits take longer than others. In addition, new patients may require more time than established ones. All this must be factored in when scheduling appointments.

Providers also have their own preferences. Some like to leave lunch hour open, while others might need a break every few patients. Finally, the facilities can have limitations. Rooms for minor surgeries may only be available certain days of the week. There might be only one electrocardiograph available, which means it must be shared among providers for their patients.

This section goes over the issues that must be considered when scheduling appointments. Each must be factored in to ensure that the appointment will work for all groups.

Patient Needs

Different kinds of patients have different kinds of needs. When scheduling appointments for new patients, the medical administrative assistant needs to request more information, so the process might take longer. Similarly, the first appointment for a new patient can be longer than one for an established patient.

The following steps should be followed when scheduling an appointment for a new patient. Medical administrative assistants usually get this information over the telephone.

- Obtain the patient's full name, birth date, address, and telephone number. Make sure the name is spelled correctly. For repeat patients, ensure that identifying information accurately matches what is on file.

- Find out if the patient has been referred by another provider. If so, you might need additional information. After the appointment, send a consultation report to the referring provider. Be sure to send a thank-you note, too.

- Request preliminary information to determine how long the appointment should be and the urgency of the need.

- Depending on the nature of the new patient's complaints, it can be necessary to ask the patient to have specific laboratory tests before the appointment.

- In some instances, the provider may request that you start building a patient medical record before the patient comes in. In other instances, it might be best to wait until after the first appointment.

- Offer the patient the first available appointment. If possible, give the individual a choice between two dates and times.

- Discuss logistics with the patient. Ask if he needs directions to the office. If so, give the exact address so the patient can get directions online. Also, provide information about parking.

- If the patient is expected to pay at the time of the visit, go over financial arrangements.

- Some medical practices mail an information packet about the office to new patients. The packet can be sent via regular mail or the Internet. The packet can be a good way to introduce a new patient to the medical staff, explain appointment policies, and describe financial arrangements.

- Before completing the call, repeat the day, date, and time of the appointment. This final step ensures that the patient has understood these details.

- If your office makes a reminder call to patients the day before their appointments, make sure to set up this service. Reminders also may be done via email or programmed telephone calls.

Established patients usually make their return appointments before leaving the office after a previous appointment. To ensure that this happens, have all patients stop by the front desk before leaving to share information or set up the next appointment. The patient's medical record should be reviewed to see if the provider has prescribed any laboratory tests or procedures.

When making in-person appointments, offer the patients a couple of choices for the day and time of their next appointments. Always give the patient an appointment card and any necessary instructions.

If an established patient chooses to make the next appointment over the phone, you don't need to go over directions or parking. If some time has passed, it's probably a good idea to verify the patient's name, address, and phone numbers; make sure an email address is on file; and recheck insurance information. Any updates should be recorded on the patient's medical record.

Providers' Preferences

When scheduling appointments, being aware of the providers' work habits and style is also important. To help you figure out the best way to accommodate the providers in the practice, think about the following questions.

- Do the providers become restless if the waiting room is not packed with patients?

- Do the providers worry if any patients are kept waiting?

- Are the providers in the building when appointments are scheduled to begin?

- Are any of the providers in the practice always late?

- Do the providers move easily from one patient to the next?

- Do any of the providers require a break after a few patients?

- Would the providers rather see fewer patients and spend more time with each one, or do they prefer seeing more patients each day?

These patterns are important to keep in mind when scheduling patients. The provider also has telephone calls to make and receive, reports to look at and dictate, meetings to attend, mail to answer, and other business responsibilities. Time must be allotted for these tasks, too.

It is also important to be aware of the availability of the nursing staff. For some examinations, such as when a male gynecologist is examining a patient, a female nurse's presence is required. If an appointment is scheduled but a nurse is not there, the appointment might need to be rescheduled. This inconveniences the patient, provider, nurse, and office staff.

One approach that helps the medical staff keep track of provider's habits is to develop a *matrix*, either online or in the appointment book. A matrix is a grid with time slots blocked out when providers are unavailable or the office is closed. For example, days off, holidays, lunch or dinner breaks, time for hospital rounds, and meetings can be blocked off on the schedule.

matrix. A grid with time slots blocked out when physicians are unavailable or the office is closed.

template. A document with a preset format that is used as a starting point so that it does not have to be recreated each time.

Computer programs usually give schedulers the option of creating a *template*. The template can be used to automatically block out times such as lunch breaks and meetings. Furthermore, the template can be used again when additional appointment pages are needed. While many providers prefer to have most of the time booked, it can be wise to set aside about 15 minutes during the day so that the provider can answer calls from patients, verify prescription calls, or answer questions.

FIGURE 1.3 *Provider's preference matrix example*

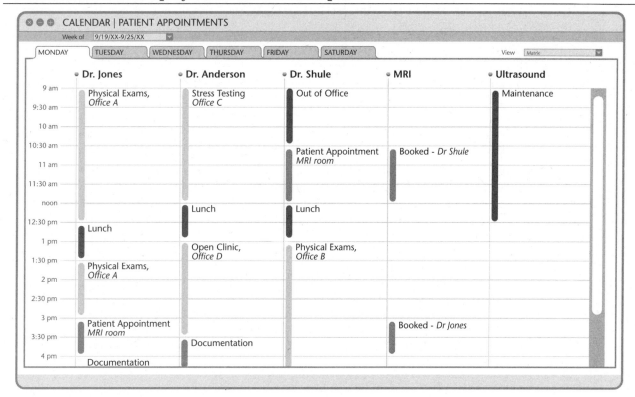

Length of Appointments

The final piece of the scheduling puzzle is knowing the amount of time needed for various office visits and procedures. Many offices have a policy and procedure manual with a list of procedures performed in the office and the timeframes typically blocked out.

There are multiple reasons for scheduling timing correctly. The most obvious is to ensure that the time of the provider, nurse, and other clinical assistants is blocked out efficiently. In addition, patients should not be kept waiting unnecessarily. Reimbursement, or payment from insurance companies, also can be linked to time requirements. Therefore, it is essential to allow enough time to complete procedures.

What are the three factors that must be considered when scheduling appointments?

ANSWER: The three factors are the patients' needs, the providers' habits and preferences, and the availability of rooms and equipment in the facility.

FOLLOWING APPOINTMENT PROTOCOLS

Every medical practice has to deal with patients who are late, cancel, or don't show up for appointments. Similarly, it's impossible for providers to avoid emergencies. Most offices have policies in place to try to deal with late or cancelled appointments and no-shows, as well as provider emergencies. This section describes the role of medical administrative assistants in implementing these policies.

Policies for Late Patients

It's not unusual for medical practices to have a few patients who are always late. When a patient is late, the medical administrative assistant should check with the physician to ensure that the patient can still be seen. One preventive strategy for dealing with this problem is to schedule these patients as the last appointment of the day. If the patient hasn't arrived by closing time, the medical staff is under no obligation to wait.

Another strategy is to ask these patients to come 30 minutes before the scheduled appointment. This gives the patients a long window for arriving, increasing the probability that they will be there when the provider is ready to see them.

Although it's important to work with all patients to ensure that they get the care they need, it's also important not to let habitually late patients disrupt the schedule. Therefore, a balance between these two concerns must be achieved.

Policies for Emergency Calls

Sometimes emergency or urgent calls come into the office. Again, the office should have procedures in place that the medical administrative assistant can follow. These procedures usually involve a *screening system* to prioritize the urgency of the call. Through screening, the medical administrative assistant can determine when the patient should be seen.

screening system. Procedures to prioritize the urgency of a call to determine when the patient should be seen.

To screen patients, it is helpful to have a list of questions available. The provider should help prepare the list, which should identify what is considered an emergency (life-threatening) or urgent (serious but not life-threatening). Among the first questions to ask are the patient's name, phone number, and location. In these situations, the patient can be referred to a hospital emergency room, or the provider might want to see the patient the same day.

If necessary, the CMAA might need to call 911 for the patient. Be sure to stay on the phone until the emergency medical technicians (EMTs) arrive. Never place an emergency call on hold.

Policies for Patients Without Appointments

It is up to the providers in the practice to develop a policy about patients who do not have appointments. If patients arrive in need of immediate attention, most providers will see them. If the patient does not need immediate care, the provider may visit with the patient briefly and then ask the medical administrative assistant to schedule an appointment. If the office policy is to turn away the patient, then the medical administrative assistant must do so.

Policies for Cancelled Appointments

When the Patient Cancels

Changing appointment times is inevitable, especially for established patients making follow-up appointments 6 months in advance. When a patient calls to reschedule an appointment, make sure the original appointment day and time have been removed from the appointment book or database. Then add the new date and time to the schedule.

If the cancellation occurs the same day as the original appointment, try to have on hand a list of patients who indicated that they would like to come in as soon as possible. Then these patients can be called to see if they are available. Cancellations of this nature should be noted on the patient's medical record, along with the reason for it. For patients who change their appointment times far enough in advance, there is no reason to note these on their records.

When the Provider Cancels

Although providers try not to cancel their appointments, sometimes events beyond their control result in this happening. If a provider is called away on an emergency or is ill, the medical administrative assistant must let the patients know. If the patient has already arrived, ask if she wants to wait or reschedule. Patients scheduled for later in the day need to be called and rescheduled. For security reasons, it is not necessary to state where the provider is or why she cancelled. Simply tell the patients that the provider is unavailable.

Policies for No-Shows

Patients sometimes fail to show up for an appointment. There are many reasons for "no-shows." Sometimes the patient simply forgets. Other patients might not have enough money to pay the provider and be staying away out of embarrassment. Still others with a serious medical condition might be in denial, so they avoid going to the doctor.

Knowing the reason for the failed appointment helps the practice deal with the patient appropriately. Call the patient to discuss the problem. If the patient's medical situation must be addressed, write a letter outlining the medical problem. Send the letter by certified mail with a return receipt request. Make sure to keep the letter in the patient's medical record in case legal documentation is ever required.

It's very important for a medical practice to have policies in place for no-shows. These policies must be clearly spelled out in the office manual.

> *certified mail.* First-class mail that also gives the mail added protection by offering insurance, tracking, and return receipt options.

Many practices follow these guidelines.

- First no-show: note it in the patient's medical record.

- Second no-show: warn the patient.

- Third no-show: consider dismissing the patient from the practice. Make sure this is done in such a way that provides legal protection for the provider.

Some providers charge fees to patients for no-shows. Because the time slot was assigned to that patient, it is ethical to charge him because no time was given to substitute another patient. In addition, the Centers for Medicare and Medicaid Services (CMS) allows providers to directly charge Medicare beneficiaries for missed appointments, as long as providers also charge non-Medicare patients for missed appointments. Many providers choose not to charge patients, but it is an option to consider.

FIGURE 1.4 *No-show documentation example*

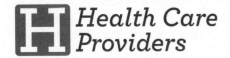

Health Care Providers

1234 Main Street
Shermer, IL 12345
1.800.555.1234

Dear Ms. Johnson,

Thank you for being a patient in our office. Sadly, we noticed that you missed your most recent appointment. If you must change an appointment, please give us at least 24 hours notice.

As your Primary Care Providers, we are very concerned about your health and safety. In reviewing your recent lab test results, it is concerning that your blood sugar levels have been averaging much higher than the normal range allows. At your last appointment, Dr. Jones noted a follow-up visit would be necessary to re-test your blood sugar levels and discuss the possibility of prescribing medication instead of a diet change approach alone. Since you missed your scheduled appointment time, we were unable to monitor your condition. Please call our office to reschedule a time for this very important follow-up visit.

You will be billed for your missed appointment. Thank you for your understanding.

Sincerely,
Health Care Providers

Strategies for Preventing and Documenting No-Shows

Most patients arrive at scheduled appointments on time, but every practice has a few who don't. In preparation for this occurrence, especially when scheduling a new patient, make sure you're aware of the office's policies on no-shows and missed or cancelled appointments.

For legal reasons, it's important to document these events in the appointment book or on the online scheduling system. This can be done using initials, such as "NS" for no-show or "MA" for missed appointment. In addition, make sure the notes are neat and legible. If the appointment book is ever brought into a court to be used as evidence, it's essential that all parties can read the documentation.

The following strategies have proven to be effective in preventing no-shows.

- *Automated Call Routing.* These calls can be made to patients scheduled for an appointment. The patient can confirm the appointment by pressing one key and cancel it by pressing another key. This tool can be used to send messages (such as reminders to get a flu vaccine) or introduce a new provider. This service also can be programmed to keep calling until the patient responds. This feature can be especially useful for patients who have a history of no-shows.

- *Appointment Cards.* These can be used to remind patients of scheduled appointments and to eliminate misunderstandings about dates and times. When giving a patient an appointment card, double-check to make sure it matches the entry in the appointment book or online system.

---

appointment cards. Used to remind patients of scheduled appointments and to eliminate misunderstandings about dates and times.

- *Confirmation Calls.* If patients have made an appointment in advance, confirmation calls are a good way to remind them to come see the doctor. For this reason, it is important to have the patients' phone numbers (work, home, and cell) handy. Before calling, make sure you know which number is the preferred one. Some patients would rather receive calls from doctors at home, not at work. Also, patients often must sign a release form stating that they agree to receive calls from their providers. This documentation should be in the patient's medical record.

- *Email Reminders.* Many computer scheduling programs can send an email reminder to patients the day before the appointment. This is an efficient way to handle reminders and frees up office staff for other tasks.

- *Mailed Reminders.* Sending reminder cards in the mail is another way to reach patients. Although this method can be somewhat time-consuming, it is worth the effort if the patient shows up for the appointment. Sometimes postcards are used instead. Then the patient can fill in the address when making the appointment. The office staff should keep the postcard in a safe place so that it is mailed at the right time.

FIGURE 1.5 *Patient reminder examples*

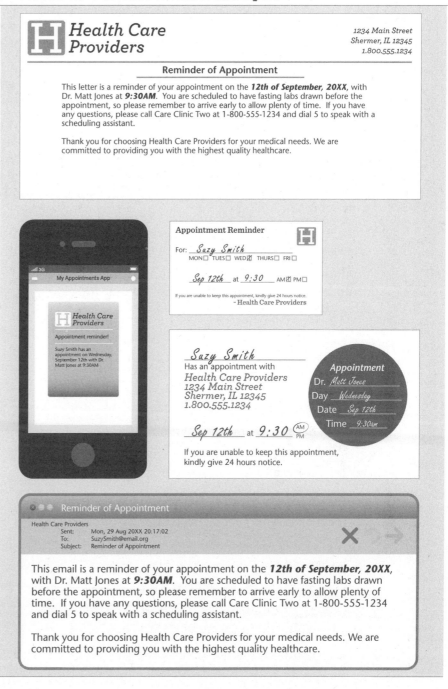

What are three strategies for preventing no-shows?

ANSWER: Strategies for preventing no-shows include automated call routing, appointment cards, and confirmation calls.

ARRANGING DIAGNOSTIC TESTING AND PROCEDURES

Medical administrative assistants often are asked to arrange outpatient diagnostic testing and procedures. Testing can include magnetic resonance imaging (MRI), computed tomography (CT) scans, x-ray evaluations, ultrasound testing, and blood tests. Possible procedures include dilation and curettage (D&C) and biopsies.

When setting up appointments for diagnostic testing or procedures, the medical administrative assistant should verify the patient's billing address and preferred method of contact, and then take the following steps.

1. Obtain a written order from the provider that describes the exact procedure to be performed. If a referral is needed, make sure you have a copy of that. This paperwork provides the necessary documentation for the test or procedure.

2. If the patient's insurance requires preauthorization, make sure to take care of this. Preauthorization involves notifying the health insurance plan that a patient needs a procedure, giving the insurance company the opportunity to determine whether the procedure is medically necessary. This will ensure that the insurance benefits are valid and will cover the patient's medical needs.

3. Make sure the patient is available on the time the test or procedure has been scheduled. If the provider needs to be there, make sure she is available as well.

4. Confirm that the diagnostic facility is a participating provider with the patient's insurance company. Then call the facility and schedule the patient's procedure or test. Remember to follow these steps.

   a. Schedule the test.

   b. Provide the patient's diagnosis and orders.

   c. Establish the date and time for the procedure.

   d. Give the patient's name, age, address, and telephone number.

   e. Provide the patient's demographic information, including identification and insurance policy numbers as well as addresses for filing claims.

   f. Determine any special instructions for the patient or special anesthesia requirements.

   g. Notify the facility of any urgency for test results.

5. Let the patient know about the arrangements. Make sure to inform the patient of the following.

   a. Name, address, and telephone number of the facility, as well as the name of the referred physician

   b. Date and time to report for the test

   c. Instructions for preparing for the test, including eating restrictions, fluid requirements, and whether medications should be taken

   d. Information about preadmission testing

   e. The need to bring a form of picture identification and his or her insurance card to the facility on the day of the procedure

   f. Whether the patient needs to pick up orders or whether they will be forwarded to the facility in advance

6. After going through the list, ask the patient to repeat the instructions. Also, remind the patient of the importance of keeping the appointment and arriving on time.

7. Have the provider review the consent form with the patient. The patient should sign the consent form, and a copy should be placed in his medical record. This process will ensure that the patient understands the risks, benefits, and alternatives to the procedure.

8. Document the information in the patient's chart. Then check the patient's status following the procedure. Make sure the patient is following the provider's postprocedure instructions. Follow up with the facility if results are not received promptly.

What steps should the medical administrative assistant take when scheduling outpatient tests or procedures?

ANSWER: The medical administrative assistant must have written documentation from the provider authorizing the procedure. In some cases, preauthorization from the patient's insurance is needed. Then schedule the test or procedure with the facility and let the patient know about the arrangements. Next, make sure the provider has reviewed the consent form with the patient, and all information has been documented on the patient's medical record. Finally, follow up with the patient after the test or procedure to ensure that she is following all postprocedure instructions. If test results are not received in a timely fashion, check up on that.

CONFIRMING FUTURE APPOINTMENTS

Following HIPAA Guidelines

When scheduling an appointment in the office, it is important to be discreet if other people are around. If any private health information is being discussed, make sure to speak in a low voice so others can't overhear the conversation.

Also, limit what you say to only what's necessary. For example, if a chemotherapy appointment is being scheduled, do not say, "Mr. Jones, we'll see you next week for your chemo appointment." Instead, say, "Mr. Jones, we'll see you next week for your regularly scheduled appointment." By leaving out reference to the type of treatment, you will go a long way toward protecting the patient's privacy.

If you're calling a patient at home and the individual does not pick up, make sure the individual has signed an agreement authorizing you to leave a message. Depending on the nature of the practice, some patients can be sensitive about messages left for others to hear.

> *Health Insurance Portability and Accountability Act (HIPAA) of 1996.* Legislation that includes Title II, the first parameters designed to protect the privacy and security of patient information.

Confirming Insurance Details

If you are scheduling a new patient, make sure that the provider is a participating member of the patient's insurance plan. Let the new patient know if there is a copayment requirement at the time services are delivered, or whether the patient will be billed after the invoice has been submitted to the insurance carrier.

When coming to the doctor, patients must bring the correct documentation. Tell the patient to bring his insurance card and photo identification to the appointment. If a referral is needed, make sure the patient brings that to the appointment as well.

> *invoice.* A document that describes items purchased or services rendered and shows the amount due.

SUMMARY

This chapter has described the importance of scheduling and the use of either hard-copy books or online systems for this purpose. It also has introduced the different strategies that can be used to schedule appointments. These include wave and modified-wave booking, double-booking, open booking, cluster booking, and open booking. Deciding on which approach works best depends on the preferences of the providers in the practice, patient needs, and facility limitations.

Most practices have an office manual describing policies for no-show, missed, cancelled, and follow-up appointments. As a medical administrative assistant, you must be knowledgeable about these practices and implement them as needed.

Another task that medical administrative assistants are often asked to do is schedule diagnostic testing and procedures. The chapter goes through step-by-step how these arrangements should be made.

The next chapter goes into more detail about taking a patient's history, verifying insurance information, and ensuring that patient records are updated regularly and completed correctly.

CHAPTER DRILL QUESTIONS

Types of Patient Scheduling

1. What are three advantages of computer scheduling?

2. When are patients scheduled in wave booking?

   a. Every 20 minutes

   b. Only in the morning

   c. At the same time each hour

   d. Intermittently throughout the day

3. How are patients scheduled in cluster or categorization booking?

   a. By age

   b. By type of insurance

   c. In alphabetical order

   d. By type of appointment

Determining Scheduling Needs

4. When scheduling appointments, what factors need to be taken into account?

5. An office schedules appointments every 20 minutes, with 30 minutes blocked off for lunch. However, the provider usually spends 30 minutes with each patient and takes 20 minutes for lunch. The waiting room is usually full. How could this office run more smoothly?

Following Appointment Protocols

6. True or False: Medical practices never charge for no-shows.

7. Why is automated call routing a good strategy for preventing no-shows?

8. A patient was scheduled for an appointment, but the doctor was called away due to an emergency. How should the medical administrative assistant handle the situation?

   a. Wait until the patient arrives and tell him what happened.

   b. If the patient is already in the office, let her wait until the doctor comes back.

   c. Try to reach the patient and let him or her know what happened. Offer alternatives for rescheduling.

   d. Call the doctor to ask him what to do.

9. Why is it important to document no-shows?

Arranging Diagnostic Procedures

10. Why is it important to get preauthorization if the patient's insurance requires you to do so?

CHAPTER DRILL ANSWERS

1. Answer: Computer systems have the capacity to display available and scheduled times, as well as length and type of appointment required and day or time preferences. Computer systems also can track future appointments.

2. **A.** INCORRECT: In wave booking, patients are scheduled at the same time each hour, not every 20 minutes.
   B. INCORRECT: In cluster or categorization booking, a practice might reserve all morning appointments for one type of visit.
   C. CORRECT: Wave booking schedules all patients at the same time each hour to create short-term flexibility each hour.
   D. INCORRECT: In open booking, or tidal wave scheduling, patients are told to come in at intermittent times. They are seen in the order in which they arrive.

3. **A.** INCORRECT: None of the scheduling types in this chapter is organized by age.
   B. INCORRECT: None of the scheduling types in this chapter is organized by type of insurance.
   C. INCORRECT: None of the scheduling types in this chapter is organized alphabetically.
   D. CORRECT: Cluster or categorization booking refers to booking different times of the day for specific kinds of patients.

4. Answer: The needs of the patient, the habits and preferences of the provider, and the capacity of the facility.

5. Answer: One way to handle this situation is to set up a meeting with the provider to go over scheduling options. Suggest reducing the time she takes for lunch and scheduling appointments every 30 minutes. Alternatively, if any patients are short appointments, you could suggest going to cluster booking, with longer appointments in the morning and shorter ones in the afternoon.

6. Answer: False. Each medical practice sets policies that meet its needs. One approach is to give patients a warning, followed by a notation in the medical record, before charging them. If those strategies don't work, providers can decide to charge these patients.

7. Answer: Automated call routing can give the patient the option to confirm or cancel the appointment. In addition, the system can be programmed to repeat the call until the patient responds.

8. **A.** INCORRECT: Do not wait until the patient arrives. Patients scheduled for later in the day need to be called and rescheduled.
   B. INCORRECT: If the patient has already arrived, ask if he wants to wait or reschedule.
   C. CORRECT: Patients scheduled for later in the day need to be called and rescheduled.
   D. INCORRECT: Call the patient to reschedule, not the doctor for advice.

9. Answer: Preauthorization is a formal approval from the insurance company that it will cover the test or procedure. If the insurance company requires this and it is not done, the patient runs the risk of having to pay the full amount for the procedure rather than having the opportunity to make other arrangements.

10. Answer: By documenting no-shows, the medical administrative assistant provides the provider with information about a patient that may warrant further action. If legal action is ever taken, the documentation can be used as evidence of patient's actions.

CHAPTER 2

Patient Intake

OVERVIEW

In any medical practice, patients are the first priority. The provider's role is to care for the patient, and the medical administrative assistant provides much-needed support. The medical administrative assistant is responsible for ensuring that all of the patient's *protected health information (PHI)* has been collected into an electronic medical record (EMR). Because electronic records are more flexible and easier to maintain, many medical practices are moving in this direction. However, some medical practices still use paper records. These, too, must be kept secure.

This chapter explains what the medical administrative assistant needs to know to accomplish these tasks. The chapter goes over how to obtain demographic and insurance information from the patient, the basics about billing and coding, and how to prepare and manage daily charts.

By the end of this chapter, you should be able to answer the following questions.

1. List three ways a medical office can accommodate patients who have vision loss.
2. Why is health insurance important?
3. True or False: If preauthorization is required but not done, the insurance carrier will not pay for the medical services provided.
4. Who is considered a guarantor?
5. What is the birthday rule?
6. What are CPT codes used to describe?
7. What is the HIPAA notice of privacy practices form?
8. Name three forms that may be found in a patient's medical record.
9. When are regular referrals needed?
10. What is included in an accurate, up-to-date medical record?

DEMOGRAPHIC INFORMATION

Collecting Basic Information

A key element of each patient's medical record is the demographics sheet. New and returning patients typically are given a form to fill out requesting the following basic information.

- Full name, spelled correctly
- Names of parents if the patient is a child
- Gender
- Date of birth
- Marital status
- Name of spouse if married
- Number of children if any
- Home address, telephone number, and email address

- Occupation
- Name of employer
- Business address and telephone number
- Employment information for spouse
- Health insurance information
- Source of referral
- Social Security number

If any questions arise, make sure you know the best way to reach the patient. Some prefer to be reached by phone, while others prefer email.

After filling out the form, patients are asked to sign it. This tells the medical staff that the patient has checked the information and it is accurate.

electronic medical record (EMR). An electronic record of health information that is created, added to, managed, and reviewed by authorized providers and staff within a single health care organization.

Collecting Basic Information from People Who Have Disabilities

Federal laws such as the Americans with Disabilities Act (ADA), which was enacted in 1990, are designed to ensure equal access to health care. For a medical office, this means that accommodations have been made so that patients who are visually impaired, have hearing loss, or have a language barrier can relay their basic information to the medical administrative assistant.

Patients who have vision loss might benefit from:

- Signage in Braille so that the office is easy to find.

- Access to important forms in large print and Braille.

- Sufficient accommodations to fill out electronic forms.

Patients who have hearing loss might benefit from:

- Obtaining their attention prior to speaking.

- Reduced background noise and auditory distractions.

- Unobstructed view of face (no masks, untrimmed mustaches, gum chewing).

Patients who have language barriers might benefit from:

- Access to necessary forms in the most common languages other than English spoken in the community.

- Knowledge of local interpreters in case that service is needed.

- Access to patient education materials in the most common languages other than English spoken in the community.

- A trained American Sign Language (ASL) interpreter to facilitate communication.

For patients who have vision loss or language barriers, the medical practice could also mail the paperwork and request that the patient bring it to the appointment. This approach requires that the patient has someone at home who can help complete the form. Before mailing out paperwork, the medical administrative assistant should verify that someone at home can help the patient with this task.

Advance Directive Forms

Another record that is often kept in the EMR is an *advance directive form*. This document spells out what kind of treatment a patient wants in the event that he can't speak for himself. Completing this form guarantees that both the provider and family know the patient's wishes if they have to make decisions on his or her behalf.

Each state has its own form for advance directives. Make sure your office has a recent version of the correct form to give to patients if needed. Later in this chapter, there is a summary of many of the forms that should be in the patient's medical record.

---

advance directive form. Document that spells out what kind of treatment a patient wants in the event that he can't speak for himself. Also known as living will.

Building the Patient Health Record

The Health Insurance Portability and Accountability Act (HIPAA) guarantees security and privacy of PHI. This includes health status, health services delivered, and payment information. PHI can refer to medical information in an electronic, paper, or verbal format.

The demographic information and advance directives should become part of the confidential EMR. The next section discusses insurance information, which also is part of each patient's health record.

protected health information (PHI). Information about health status or health care that can be linked to a specific individual.

Name three types of information that fall under the heading "demographics."

ANSWER: Three types of information under the heading "demographics" are name, address, and marital status.

INSURANCE INFORMATION

The purpose of health insurance is to help individuals and families pay for their medical care. Health insurance is protection against financial losses because of illness or injury. Think of insurance as financial support for medical needs, hospitalization, medically necessary diagnostic tests and procedures, and many kinds of preventive services.

Part of the medical administrative assistant's job is to obtain information about the insurance coverage of each patient. It's important to have this information in the EHR so that the office staff knows which routine and special procedures and services are covered by insurance. Insurance coverage also protects both the patient and provider against unexpected medical care costs.

electronic health record (EHR). An electronic record of health-related information about a patient that conforms to nationally recognized interoperability standards that can be created, managed, and reviewed by authorized providers and staff from more than one health care organization.

To ensure that the right information is on file, the medical administrative assistant must complete the following tasks.

- Verify the policyholder and the patient's eligibility for insurance with the carrier. This can be done electronically. When communicating with someone from the insurance carrier's office, be sure to get the name, title, and phone number of that individual.

- Confirm the benefits available, services that are excluded, and whether special authorization is needed to refer patients to specialists or perform certain services or procedures. If you are verifying coverage for an established patient, make sure that there have been no changes to the patient's coverage.

- When the patient comes to the office, ask to see her insurance card and verify the effective date the insurance began. Then photocopy both sides to ensure that the information is correct. Also, copayments (see below) and emergency departments might be listed on the back. Finally, ask to see photo identification, such as a driver's license, to verify the patient's identity.

FIGURE 2.1 *Patient insurance card example*

HEALTH INSURANCE EXAMPLE COMPANY	*Preferred Benefits Program*	
Caroline D. Moore ID #: ABC1234567890 Suffix: 00	Effective Date: **12 July 20XX**	
Group #: 98765432 Plan: PPO	Emergency Room Urgent Care Office Visit Specialist	$150.00 $50.00 $25.00 $50.00
Customer Service:1.800.555.9876	*123 Office Parkway	Fettle, MO 54321*	

- Many insurance plans require a *copayment*, or fees collected at the time of services. Copayments usually range up to $45 for office visits and $75 for specialists. Patients also may have coinsurance, or a percentage of the fees that they share with the insurance company. An 80/20 (80% to the insurance carrier and 20% to the patient) is a common arrangement. In addition, any services not covered by the insurance company typically are passed on to the patient. Before the patient can be billed, however, he must sign an agreement to assume the financial risk. The form to use is discussed later in this chapter.

- Document the information collected in the patient's medical record and on a Verification of Benefits form. (*Note: The next section includes discussion of forms that must be signed by the patient.*)

- Follow the billing department's policy for explaining the plan's requirements and possible restrictions, or non-covered items. The explanation also may include the patient's responsibility in meeting billing requirements.

- Explain the referral process to the patient. If referrals are required, make sure that he or she understands that without a referral, the patient is responsible for paying for the provider's services.

Why is it important to verify a patient's insurance?

ANSWER: Verifying insurance ensures that the patient is covered and determines the benefits that will be paid for routine and special procedures and services. Verification also protects the provider and patient against unexpected medical care costs.

Precertification and Preauthorization

Before certain procedures can be performed or a patient hospitalized, many insurance companies require precertification or preauthorization, usually within 24 hours. Many managed care systems require preauthorization for a patient to be referred to a specialist. They also have requirements about which laboratories patients can go to for certain tests. Knowing when to get preauthorization is an important part of the medical administrative assistant's job. If this is not done, insurance claims will be denied.

Primary and Secondary Coverage

While most people have one insurance plan, it is possible to be covered by two. For example, one insurance plan might be an insurance plan offered through an employer, while the second could be Medicare.

When the patient is the same as the insured, the patient is also referred to as the *guarantor*. That insurance is considered the patient's primary insurance. Typically, adults are their own guarantors, with exceptions for cases such as accidents caused by a third party or workers' compensation claims. If the patient is also covered by a second policy, that is referred to as the secondary insurance. Typically, the primary insurance pays first. If the service was a covered benefit under the second plan, then it pays the balance.

guarantor. Person or entity responsible for the remaining payment of services after insurance has paid.

In addition, CMS allows providers to directly charge Medicare beneficiaries for missed appointments, as long as the providers also charge non-Medicare patients for missed appointments.

Birthday Rule

This informal procedure has been widely adopted by the insurance industry. It applies to dependent children whose parents have more than one insurance policy. Under the birthday rule, the health plan of the parent whose birthday comes first in the calendar year is designated as the primary plan. It doesn't matter how old the parent is or which parent is older; the issue is the date of birth and which comes first.

> *birthday rule.* The health plan of the parent whose birthday comes first in the calendar year is designated as the primary plan.

There are some exceptions to the birthday rule.

- If both parents have the same birthday, the health plan that has covered the parent the longest is considered the primary plan.

- If the parents are separated or divorced, the health plan of the parent who has custody of children is considered the primary plan. If one spouse has insurance under a group plan and the other spouse has an individual plan, the group plan is primary.

- If one parent is employed and has a health insurance plan and the other parent has insurance through a former employer (such as through the Consolidated Omnibus Budget Reconciliation Act, or COBRA) and the children are listed as dependents on both plans, the plan of the active employee is the primary plan.

CODING SYSTEMS

The following coding systems are used to report diagnoses, procedures, and services.

> *Healthcare Common Procedure Coding System (HCPCS).* A group of codes and descriptors used to represent health care procedures, supplies, products, and services.

- ICD-10-CM (diagnoses for all providers)

- ICD-10-PCS (hospital inpatient procedures only)

- CPT (outpatient procedures and services, including physician offices)

- HCPCS Level II (outpatient procedures and services, including physician offices)

ICD-10-CM and ICD-10-PCS

ICD-10-CM

ICD-10-CM disease and injury codes contain up to seven alphanumeric characters, such as T82.120S (Displacement of cardiac electrode, sequela). Assignment requires the interpretation of coding conventions (e.g., Code also, Excludes 1). The first character of an ICD-10-CM code is always a letter, and codes that contain four or more characters require the use of a decimal. The placeholder "x" is used when a seventh character is required but there is no fifth and/or sixth character, such as T14.8xxA (Other injury of unspecified body region, initial encounter).

ICD-10-CM contains an (1) Index to Diseases and Injuries, which includes a Neoplasm Table, Table of Drugs and Chemicals, and an Index to External Causes; and a (2) Tabular List of Diseases and Injuries. Main terms in the index are boldfaced, and subterms are indented. When using the ICD-10-CM index to locate a code, the tabular list must be reviewed to validate accuracy of code assignment.

ICD-10-PCS

ICD-10-PCS procedure codes contain seven alphanumeric characters (using letters A-H, J-N, and P-Z), such as 0DTJ0ZZ (Resection of Appendix, Open Approach). No decimal is used in ICD-10-PCS codes, and letters I and O are not used (because they could be confused with numbers 1 and 0). ICD-10-PCS contains an (1) Index and (2) Tables. Main terms in the index are boldfaced, and subterms are indented. When using the ICD-10-PCS index to locate a procedure, the appropriate table must be used to "build a code" (e.g., index main term "Appendectomy" directs the coder to table 0DTJ to locate the fifth through seventh characters, resulting in 0DTJ0ZZ for an open approach or 0DTJ4ZZ for a percutaneous endoscopic approach).

ICD-10-PCS procedures are organized into 17 sections, which include:

- 0 Medical and Surgical
- 1 Obstetrics
- 2 Placement
- 3 Administration
- 4 Measurement and Monitoring
- 5 Extracorporeal or Systemic Assistance and Performance
- 6 Extracorporeal or Systemic Therapies
- 7 Osteopathic
- 8 Other Procedures
- 9 Chiropractic
- B Imaging
- C Nuclear Medicine
- D Radiation Therapy
- F Physical Rehabilitation and Diagnostic Audiology
- G Mental Health
- H Substance Abuse Treatment
- X New Technology

The first character of an ICD-10-PCS code always corresponds to the section where the procedure is classified. The second through seventh characters have specific meanings, which are unique to each section.

Healthcare Common Procedure Coding System (HCPCS)

HCPCS is a group of codes and descriptors used to represent healthcare procedures, supplies, products, and services. HCPCS is divided into two levels. Level I is the Current Procedure Terminology (CPT) codes, which are maintained by the American Medical Association (AMA). Level II codes, also called National Codes, are maintained by CMS. Each of these levels is described in the next sections.

reimbursement. Payment from insurance companies.

modifiers. Added information or changed description of procedures and services, and are a part of valid CPT or HCPCS codes.

HCPCS Level I

CPT is a uniform code that accurately describes and reports medical, surgical, and diagnostic services and procedures. Providers use CPT codes for hospital inpatient and outpatient services and for those performed in other facilities. Because the CPT code set was adapted for Medicare, it is referred to as HCPCS Level I in the coding and reimbursement communities.

CPT codes are divided into Category I, II, and III groupings.

Category I CPT codes are five-digit codes and two-digit modifiers. Modifiers use both Level I and II HCPCS to change the code description. For example, modifier 50 is used to describe a bilateral procedure. Modifier 22 indicates that a procedure was decreased or limited. Category I CPT codes primarily cover providers' services but are used for hospital outpatient coding, too. According to the AMA, *Category II codes* were designed to serve as supplemental tracking codes that can be used for performance measurement. Although these codes are optional, they do provide more information about a patient's visit and treatment plan.

Category III codes are used for temporary coding for new technology and services that have not met the requirements needed to be added to the main section of the CPT book. These codes are not optional. They should be used to report procedures performed.

Codes in this section are evaluated and added every 6 months. As Category I codes are created to describe new procedures, the temporary Category III codes are deleted. After about 5 years, if the Category III codes are not used, they are deleted.

HCPCS Level II

HCPCS Level II codes were established to report services, supplies, and procedures not represented in CPT. These codes begin with a letter from A-V, followed by four numbers. The letter identifies the code section and type of service or supply coded. Descriptions identify items or services, not specific brand names. For example, A codes cover ambulance and transportation services; medical and surgical supplies; and administrative, miscellaneous, and investigational services and supplies.

HCPCS also allows for modifiers, which can be used for all levels of HCPCS codes, including CPT codes. They add more specific information to what's referenced in the main code. For example, AA codes stand for anesthesia services performed by an anesthesiologist and E1 codes refer to procedures done to the upper left eyelid.

What are the two kinds of coding systems and how are they used?

ANSWER: Clinical coding systems, such as the International Classification of Diseases, Tenth Revision, Clinical Modification (ICD-10-CM) track a patient's diagnosis and clinical history. Procedural coding systems, such as Current Procedural Terminology (CPT) codes and the Healthcare Common Procedure Coding System (HCPCS), are used to report provider services for the purpose of reimbursement.

ENSURING COMPLETION OF FORMS

Throughout this chapter, many different kinds of forms have been mentioned. These documents are important because they track many aspects of the patient's care and insurance: medical benefits, how a patient wants providers to be paid, and treatment preferences in the event of a terminal illness, to name a few. It is the job of the medical administrative assistant to make sure the proper forms have been distributed, signed, and filed in the patient's record.

The following section describes some of the forms typically kept in a patient's file. Samples of each form have also been included.

Health history form. This is a lengthy form that asks patients to list any illnesses or surgeries they have had, their family history, medications taken, chronic health issues, allergies, and other providers they have consulted.

Notice of privacy practices. Under HIPAA, medical practices are not allowed to release information unless patients first sign a notice of privacy practices form. This form explains what's in a patient's medical record, the patient's health information rights (e.g., request a restriction on certain uses and disclosures of information, obtain a paper copy of the notice, and amend health record requests in writing), and the medical practice's responsibilities to the patient.

Consent to release information. Once the patient has read the notice of privacy practices, he will be asked to sign a HIPAA-compliant consent to disclose information to other health care professionals involved in the patient's care. The purpose of allowing disclosure is so the patient's providers and other health care professionals can coordinate diagnosis and treatment.

FIGURE 2.2 *Consent to release information*

Health Care Providers

1234 Main Street
Shermer, IL 12345
1.800.555.1234

Patient Consent to the Use and Disclosure of Health Information for Treatment, Payment, or Health Care Operations

I understand that as part of my health care, the practice originates and maintains paper and/or electronic records describing my health history, symptoms, examination and test results, diagnoses, treatment, and any plans for future care or treatment. I understand that this information serves as:
- A basis for planning my care and treatment,
- A means of communication among professionals who contribute to my care,
- A source of information for applying my diagnosis and treatment information to my bill,
- A means by which a third-party payer can verify that services billed were actually provided
- A tool for routine health care operations, such as assessing quality.

I have been provided the opportunity to review the "Notice of Patient Privacy Information Practices" that provides a more complete description of information uses and disclosures. I understand that I have the following rights:
- The right to review the "Notice" prior to acknowledging this consent,
- The right to restrict or revoke the use or disclosure of my health information for other uses or purposes, and
- The right to request restrictions as to how my health information may be used or disclosed to carry out treatment, payment, or health care operations.

<u>Restrictions</u>
I request the following restrictions to the use or disclosure of my health information:

_____
_____
_____
_____

May discuss treatment, payment, or health care operation with the following persons:

_____
_____
_____
_____

I understand that as part of treatment, payment, or health care operations, it may become necessary to disclose health information to another entity, i.e., referrals to other health care providers, labs, and/or individuals or agencies as permitted or required by state or federal law.

I fully understand and accept the information provided by this consent.

_____   _____   _____
Signatue   Printed name   Date

Authorization to release medical records. If a provider needs medical records from another provider, the patient must sign a medical release form. Before the patient signs it, make sure he understands that the medical facility will now have the authority to share medical information. After the patient signs the form, make a copy for the patient's file. Before sending the form to the facility, make sure a current privacy policy document is on file.

Patient financial responsibility form. This form confirms that the patient is responsible for payments to the provider. It also states that insurance carriers can mail payments directly to the provider. The form goes on to state that any payments not covered by insurance must be paid by the patient.

Assignment of benefits (AOB) form. This form authorizes health insurance benefits to be sent directly to providers. AOB forms are only valid for facilities in the United States. The form clearly states that if the insurance does not cover the claim, the insured individual is responsible.

The following set of forms explains the options patients have for expressing their wishes at the end of life.

Advance directives. An advance directives form outlines the patient's wishes for care at end of life. Most states have forms that can be found online and used for this purpose. The form lays out whether the patient wants steps taken to prolong life, pain management preferences, choice of provider, and whether the patient wants her organs donated. For this form to be valid, it must be signed by the patient and two adult witnesses, or signed in front of a notary.

Living will. A limited version of advance directives, this form states that a patient does not desire to have any treatments to prolong life. This form also has a place where the patient can name a health surrogate, who is legally designated to act on his or her behalf. Each state also has a copy of this form, which can be found online.

DNR form. Often accompanied by a living will, a do not resuscitate (DNR) form states that the patient does not want to be revived if there are no signs of life. Although patients often think that a living will is sufficient, medics will perform CPR unless a DNR is in the patient's chart.

health history form. Form that asks patients to list any illnesses or surgeries they have had, family history, medications taken, chronic health issues, allergies, and other physicians they consulted.

Notice of Privacy Practices. Document informing a patient of when and how their PHI can be used.

consent. A patient's permission.

patient financial responsibility form. Form that confirms that the patient is responsible for payments to the provider.

assignment of benefits (AOB) form. Form that authorizes health insurance benefits to be sent directly to providers.

living will. Document that spells out what kind of treatment a patient wants in the event that he can't speak for himself. Also known as advance directive.

DNR form. Form that states that the patient does not want to be revived after experiencing a heart episode or other kind of life-threatening event.

Why do providers request that patients sign consent to release information forms?

ANSWER: These forms allow providers to legally request needed information from other health care professionals who might have treated the patient. The ability to find out more about the patient's medical history improves the overall quality of care.

PREPARING ENCOUNTER FORMS

After seeing a patient, the provider typically fills out an *encounter form*, previously called superbills. Paper versions of these forms usually have a white top sheet, a yellow sheet, and a pink sheet.

encounter form. A document used to collect data about elements of a patient visit that can become part of a patient record or be used for management purposes.

With the increase in EHR, fewer clinics are using the three-part encounter form. Most insurance claims are sent electronically. A patient needing a copy of the encounter for insurance will be given a printed copy. In some cases, the patient can print her own from an online patient portal provided by the provider.

The encounter form includes information about the patient, such as the person's name, account number, and previous balance. Current charges and payments for the visit are added after the provider sees the patient. The provider also may indicate when the patient should return for a visit.

After receiving the encounter form, the medical administrative assistant should verify the information in the form and schedule the next appointment. She can then write the date and time on the patient's copy of the form.

Processing Referrals

After seeing a patient, the provider may decide that the patient needs to see a specialist. It is up to the medical administrative assistant to complete the referral form. The form typically includes information about the patient's insurance. It is sent to the patient's insurance carrier to inform the carrier of the patient's condition and, to request preauthorization, or approval, from the insurance carrier if necessary.

When approving the request, the insurance carrier provides a verification or authorization number and confirms the specific number of procedures, services, or treatment sessions allowed. The carrier also provides authorization for referral to a specialist. There are three kinds of referrals.

regular referral. When a physician decides that a patient needs to see a specialist.

urgent referral. When an urgent, but not life-threatening, situation occurs, requiring that the referral be taken care of quickly.

stat referral. Needed in an emergency situation, and can be approved immediately over the telephone after the utilization review has approved the faxed document.

- A *regular referral* is when the provider decides that the patient needs to see a specialist. This process usually takes 3 to 10 working days for review and approval. It is the most common type of referral.

- An *urgent referral* is when an urgent, but not life-threatening, situation occurs, requiring that the referral be taken care of quickly. This process usually takes about 24 hours.

- A *stat referral* is needed in an emergency situation, and can be approved immediately over the telephone after the utilization review has approved the faxed document.

TABLE 2.1 *Referral examples*

SPECIALIST	REFERRAL NEEDS
Gastroenterologist	Esophagogastroduodenoscopy (EGD), colonoscopy
Cardiologist	Holter monitor, cardiac stress test
Dermatologist	Removal of skin cancer, allergy testing
Orthopedic surgeon	Hip replacement, knee arthroscopy

Back-Office Procedures

The "back office" generally refers to the clinical side of the practice or facility. Although the medical administrative assistant does not need to have expertise on all clinical details, it is important to have a basic knowledge of procedures performed in the back office, as well as diagnosis and procedure codes associated with those procedures. The medical administrative assistant must be able to quickly recognize the procedure or condition for a given patient based on assigned codes, which are explained earlier in this chapter. Back office procedures can also refer to administrative work that occurs away from patients, including ensuring that the correct information is in the patient's file, processing forms, processing referrals, and filing the encounter form.

What information is on the encounter form?

ANSWER: The encounter form includes the patient's name, account number, previous balance, and when the patient needs to come back.

PREPARING DAILY CHARTS

Creating and keeping medical records, or charts, up-to-date and filed accurately is one of the most important jobs of the medical administrative assistant. This job is ongoing. Each day, patients are seen, and changes are made to their records. Reports can come in from laboratories or other facilities. The medical administrative assistant must make sure the provider sees those as well.

Filing Patients' Charts

The following steps must be followed to ensure that charts are maintained and filed correctly.

- After all patients have left, check their files to make sure all new information has been recorded. Also, make sure the entries are clear and easy to read. Ensure that all records are matched to the correct patient.

- Give the providers all reports of abnormal findings to read and initial so that action can be taken. After the reports have been returned, file them in the correct section of the patient's chart. Always make sure that the name of the patient matches the new information added to his or her chart.

- If the policy in your office is to show the provider all reports—normal and abnormal—make sure to do so.

- Patients' records should *not* leave the office. A provider's pocket call record can be used for outside calls. The information can be transferred to the chart in the office. Notes about any missed appointments or refusals to cooperate with instructions should be made.

- After all the records have been reviewed for the day, place them in a file tray and lock them up for the night if there is not time to file them. Do not leave the files out where anyone can see them, especially if a cleaning service comes in.

- The next morning, index the histories for filing. Attach extra reports and information sheets. Make sure they are attached permanently; don't just drop the forms into the folders. Now the records are ready for filing.

- To make sure all the information about each patient is put in the correct file, develop an easy-to-use filing system. It can be color-coded or a numeric system. This system will also ensure that providers are given the correct chart before meeting and examining a patient.

Retrieving Patients' Charts

In order to be able to find each patient's record quickly, an efficient filing system must be in place. Most medical offices use the following classification system.

- *Active files* are the files of patients currently receiving treatment.

- *Inactive files* are the files of patients whom the provider has not seen for 6 months or longer. When these patients come back for a visit, their files should be put back among the active files.

- *Closed files* are those of patients who have died, moved away, or terminated their relationship with the provider for another reason.

Charts for patients in the hospital may be kept in a special section and then put back in the active file when each patient is discharged. Similarly, a system should be in place for easy, regular transfer of files from active to inactive status, or possibly destruction. The process of moving a file from active to inactive status is called *purging*. One way to identify files for purging is to stamp the outside of each file with the date a patient was last seen or use a sticker with this information. Then it is easy to see when a chart should become inactive. This approach is called the *perpetual transfer method*.

active files. Section of medical charts for patients currently receiving treatment.

inactive files. Section of medical charts for patients the provider has not seen for 6 months or longer.

closed files. Section of medical charts for patients who have died, moved away, or terminated their relationship with the physician.

purging. The process of moving a file from active to inactive status.

perpetual transfer method. Identifying files for purging by marking the outside of the file.

Elements of Medical Records

Throughout this chapter, different elements of the medical record have been described. Because the records for individual patients are the most important ones in the office, all of their components are listed here. Different facilities organize medical information in varying ways, and these elements may be sections of a medical chart or included as parts of other records. The medical administrative assistant is responsible for keeping track of these records.

- *Personal demographics.* This information includes basic facts about the patient, such as name, sex, date of birth, name of spouse, number of children, home address, telephone number, email address, and occupation.

- *Personal and medical history.* This includes information about past illnesses or surgeries, physical defects (congenital or acquired), and information about daily health habits. Stickers can be used on the front of the medical record to indicate allergies, advance directives, and other important information.

- *Family history.* This includes the physical condition of various members of the patient's family, illnesses or diseases family member had, and a record of the causes of death. Much of this information is focused on the immediate family.

- *Patient's social history.* This includes information about lifestyle, such as drinking, smoking, and illegal drug use. Marital information also can be put here.

- *Patient's chief complaint.* This is a concise summary of the patient's symptoms, including nature and duration of pain (if any), when the symptoms were first noticed, remedies the patient may have tried, whether the patient had this problem before, and any treatments used for this problem.

- *Physical examination findings and laboratory and radiology reports.* The results of the physical examination, as well as the findings from other tests.

- *Diagnosis.* Based on all the information gathered, the provider makes a diagnosis. If there is some uncertainty about the diagnosis, it may be labeled *provisional diagnosis.* A *differential diagnosis* is the process of weighing the probability that other diseases are the cause of the problem. For example, a differential diagnosis of a rhinitis, or a runny nose, could indicate a cause of allergies, the common cold, or even abuse of drugs or nasal decongestants.

  provisional diagnosis. A temporary or working diagnosis.

  differential diagnosis. The process of weighing the probability that other diseases are the cause of the problem.

- *Treatment.* The provider's suggested treatment. On each subsequent visit, the date must be entered, along with information about the patient's condition and the results of treatment, based on the provider's observations. Notes about medications and instructions given, as well as the patient's own progress report, should be added as well. Home visits, hospitalizations, and admission and discharge dates all should be included. These progress notes keep the file up-to date.

- *Termination.* When the treatment for a particular problem has been completed, the provider should make sure to include this information.

Planning Ahead

At the end each day, it is a good idea to look over the appointments scheduled for the next day. Then review the medical records for scheduled patients. If laboratory tests or other procedures were scheduled, determine whether the results have come in. If so, put them in the patient's medical record. If a patient is scheduled for a particular procedure, make sure everything that is needed is available.

These steps can help make the next day go smoothly. It will be easier to retrieve the files needed for the day and to be prepared to greet each patient appropriately. They also will save time during another busy day.

SUMMARY

This chapter has covered many tasks of medical administrative assistants. These include how to obtain patient demographics, verify insurance information, collect appropriate forms and make sure they are complete, process referrals and prepare encounter forms, and keep track of each patient's medical record.

The next chapter focuses on different ways to file medical records, collect copayments and create billing statements, and make sure mail is sorted and distributed correctly. Performing these tasks well will help keep the office running efficiently.

CHAPTER DRILL QUESTIONS

Demographic Information

1. List three ways a medical office can accommodate patients who have vision loss.

Insurance Information

2. Why is health insurance important?

3. True or False: If preauthorization is required but not done, the insurance carrier will not pay for the medical services provided.

4. Who is considered a guarantor?

   a. The patient's employer

   b. The insurance carrier

   c. The provider

   d. The patient who also is the owner of the primary insurance plan.

5. What is the birthday rule?

Coding Systems

6. What are CPT codes used to describe?

   a. Supplies used during surgery

   b. Type of insurance a patient has

   c. Services provided by providers

   d. Payments received from third-party payers

Ensuring Completion of Forms

7. What is the HIPAA notice of privacy practices form?

8. Name three forms that may be found in a patient's medical record.

Preparing Encounter Forms

9. When are regular referrals needed?

   a. A patient wants to change providers.

   b. A provider decides that the patient needs to see a specialist.

   c. When coding providers' notes.

   d. When answering questions from insurance companies.

Preparing Daily Charts

10. What is included in an accurate, up-to-date medical record?

    a. Only demographic information

    b. Patient history but no insurance information

    c. Only laboratory reports

    d. All information relevant to patient medical care and insurance

CHAPTER DRILL ANSWERS

1. Answer: Possible answers include having signage in Braille so the patient can find the office; having documents in Braille and large print; and having modifications built into the computer if the patient is asked to complete any forms electronically.

2. Answer: Health insurance is important because if serves as protection against financial losses due to illness or injury. Insurance provides financial support for medical needs, hospitalization, medically necessary diagnostic tests and procedures, and many kinds of preventive services.

3. Answer: True. Before certain procedures can be performed or a patient hospitalized, many insurance companies require precertification or preauthorization. If this is not done, insurance claims will be denied.

4. **A.** INCORRECT: The patient's employer is not the guarantor.

   B. INCORRECT: The insurance carrier is not the guarantor.

   C. INCORRECT: The provider is not the guarantor.

   D. CORRECT: When the patient is the same as the insured, the patient is also referred to as the guarantor.

5. Answer: The birthday rule applies to dependent children whose parents have more than one insurance policy. Under the birthday rule, the health plan of the parent whose birthday comes first in the calendar year is designated as the primary plan.

6. **A.** INCORRECT: HCPCS Level II codes were established to report services, supplies, and procedures not represented in CPT.

   B. INCORRECT: CPT codes do not document types of insurance.

   C. CORRECT: Providers use CPT codes for hospital inpatient and outpatient services.

   D. INCORRECT: CPT codes do not document payments received.

7. Answer: Under HIPAA, medical practices are not allowed to release information unless patients first sign a notice of privacy practices form. This form explains what's in a patient's medical record, the patient's health information rights (e.g., request a restriction on certain uses and disclosures of information, obtain a paper copy of the notice, and amend, health record requests in writing), and the medical practice's responsibilities to the patient.

8. Answer: Examples of forms found in a patient's medical record include consent to release information, patient financial responsibility form, and advance directives.

9. **A.** INCORRECT: Referrals are not needed when a patient changes providers.

   B. CORRECT: A regular referral is when the provider decides that the patient needs to see a specialist.

   C. INCORRECT: Referrals are not needed when coding providers' notes.

   D. INCORRECT: Referrals are not needed when answering questions from insurance companies.

10. **A.** INCORRECT: Medical records include more than just demographic information.

    B. INCORRECT: Medical records include both patient history and insurance information.

    C. INCORRECT: Medical records include more than just laboratory reports.

    D. CORRECT: Medical records contain all information relevant to patient medical care and insurance.

CHAPTER 3
Office Logistics

OVERVIEW

In a busy medical practice, the key to success is organization. Organization involves keeping files—both paper and electronic—in order, with updates made regularly and filing done so that the files are easy to find and access. It also means having efficient systems in place for determining patients' fees after factoring in deductibles, copayments, and coinsurance, as well as following the basic rules of bookkeeping.

This chapter covers these important parts of managing office logistics. It also goes over what the medical administrative assistant needs to know about sorting and delivering mail and using different classes of mail offered by the U.S. Postal Service, such as first-class, registered, and certified, as well as private companies such as FedEx.

By the end of this chapter, you should be able to answer the following questions.

1. What are three filing systems used for paper files?
2. True or False: Cross-reference sheets are needed for numeric filing systems.
3. What is involved in a terminal numbering system?
4. Why is it important to use a good system when filing charts?
5. What is the difference between a copayment and coinsurance?
6. True or False: The allowable amount is not taken into account when determining how much the patient owes.
7. What is a day sheet?
8. A provider bought a new piece of equipment for $2,000. The office put down $500 and has a balance of $1,500. What part of the equation is the provider's assets?
9. What is the difference between an EHR and an EMR?
10. When should registered mail be used?

FILING MEDICAL RECORDS

As discussed in Chapter 2, building the patient's confidential medical record is one of the most important parts of the medical administrative assistant's job. Not only does it involve gathering the right information and keeping it updated, it also means maintaining the filing system established by the office. Some offices use paper files; others use electronic files; and still others use a combination of both.

This section discusses different filing systems. It begins with paper files, followed by information about electronic health records (EHRs) and electronic medical records (EMRs).

Filing Systems for Paper Files

Generally, medical practices tend to use three basic filing systems.

- Alphabetic by name

- Numeric

- Subject

Patients' records are usually filed by name or using one of several numeric systems. Subject filing is reserved for business records, correspondence, and information related to a specific topic, such as facility management and maintenance.

Alphabetic Filing by Name

This is the oldest, simplest, and most commonly used system. It is also the preferred system in most providers' offices. Alphabetic filing by name is referred to as a *direct filing system* because the only information needed for accurate filing and retrieval is the patient's name.

However, it does have some limitations.

direct filing system. System in which the only information needed for filing and retrieval is a patient's name.

- The correct spelling of the patient's name must be known.

- As the number of files increases, more space is needed for each section of the alphabet. File folders might then need to be shifted periodically to allow for expansion.

- As the files expand, more time is needed for filing and retrieval because more files have to be searched before finding the right one. Color-coding can help reduce the search time. Color-coding also helps make it easier to spot misfiled folders.

Alphabetic Color-Coding

When combining color-coding with the alphabetic system, five different-colored files might be used. Each color represents a segment of the alphabet. The second letter of the patient's last name determines the color. Another approach is to use two sets of 13 colors: one set for letters A-M and a second set of the same colors on a different background for letters N-Z.

Self-adhesive, colored letter blocks with either two or three letters in the specific colors can be purchased in rolls. The color blocks with the appropriate letters should be placed on the index tab of the folder, along with the patient's full name. The letters are in pairs so that they can be seen from either side of the chart. Strong, easily differentiated colors are used, creating a band of color in the files that makes it easier to see misplaced folders.

Numeric Filing

Most large clinics and hospitals use some form of numeric filing, often combined with color-coding. There are multiple schools of thought about when to use numeric filing. Some experts recommend using it only if there are more than 5,000 charts. Others recommend this approach for more than 10,000 charts, or for more than 15,000 charts. Still other experts recommend this system over all others.

Numeric filing is an example of an indirect filing system. This means that it requires the use of an alphabetic *cross-reference* to find a given file. This is a disadvantage, but there are many clear advantages to this approach.

cross-reference. Reference to corresponding information in a separate location.

- It allows unlimited expansion without periodic shifting of folders, and shelves usually fill up evenly.

- It provides additional confidentiality to the chart.

- It saves time retrieving and refiling records, so these tasks can be done quickly. For example, it is obvious that 540 falls between 539 and 541. An alphabetic system usually requires a longer search, even with color-coding.

What are two advantages of a numeric filing system?

ANSWER: A numeric filing system allows unlimited expansion without periodic shifting of folders and provides additional confidentiality to the chart.

There are several types of numeric systems.

- *Straight or consecutive numeric system.* Under this system, patients are given consecutive numbers as they join the practice. This is the simplest numeric system and works well for up to 10,000 records. One downside of this approach is that it is time-consuming, and the chance for error is greater when documents with five or more digits are filed.

- *Terminal digit system.* Patients are also assigned consecutive numbers, but the digits in the number are usually separated into groups of twos or threes. They are then read in groups from right to left instead of from left to right. The records are filed backward in groups. For example, all files ending in "00" are grouped together first, followed by those ending in "01"; the system continues in this fashion. Next, the files are grouped by their middle digits so that the "00 22s" come before the "01 22s."

- *Middle digit filing.* This system of filing begins with the middle digits. They are followed by the first digit and then by the terminal digits.

TABLE 3.1 *More about cross-referencing*

A cross-referencing system does not have to be complicated. Follow these steps to develop a simple, workable system.

1. Identify the label for the primary file.

2. Make a file to be used as the primary medical file.

3. Identify one or more other places where information about the patient can be found.

4. For the alternative filings, make a cross-reference sheet, card, or chart that lists the primary reference and states where it can be found.

Numeric Color-Coding

The way color-coding is used in numeric filing is that the numbers 0 through 9 are assigned different colors. In a terminal digit system, the colors for the last two numbers are put on the tab. For example, if the number 1 is red and the number 5 is yellow, all files with numbers ending in 15 form a red and yellow band.

Subject Filing

Typically used for general correspondence, subject filing can be alphabetic or alphanumeric, such as A 1-1, A 1-2, etc. The main problem with this approach is that it can be difficult to decide where to file a document. For this reason, many papers need to be accompanied by a cross-referencing sheet. For example, when organizing correspondence, all papers dealing with a particular subject should be filed together in chronological order. Then the subject headings should be placed on the tabs of the folders and filed alphabetically.

Organizing Charts

So far, the chapter has discussed the importance of filing folders efficiently so that they are easy to find. However, the internal organization of the chart is equally important. To locate information, it needs to be arranged in a logical way.

One way to do this is by organizing the information by topic. That means putting all similar information in the same place.

Below are some categories that you can use to organize medical charts.

- Personal and family history
- Clinical progress, including notes from the provider
- Laboratory results
- Medications prescribed
- Insurance information
- Referrals
- Legal documents, such as advance directives
- HIPAA-related documents

The categories vary from practice to practice. For example, a physical therapy office will have categories for therapy prescribed, progress, and discharge summary.

Scanning Documents

Sometimes medical administrative assistants have to use scanners to put relevant information, such as photos, text, or illustrations, into a more computer-friendly format. This involves putting the pages into a scanner, saving them onto the computer, and then incorporating them into a document. Some scanners can collect specific notes from printed text, serving the function of a highlighter.

In some instances, documents are scanned and sent by email. Then the medical administrative assistant must know how to download those documents and file them in the proper place. Also, older information from patients' records may be scanned and stored so the paper files can be purged, or destroyed.

Difference Between EHRs and EMRs

There has been some confusion about the terms *electronic health records (EHRs)* and *electronic medical records (EMRs)*. For this reason, the National Alliance for Health Information Technology (NAHIT) established clear definitions for each term.

The EHR is an electronic record of health-related information about a patient that conforms to nationally recognized interoperability standards that can be created, managed, and reviewed by authorized providers and staff from *more than one health care organization*.

The EMR is an electronic record of health information that is created, added to, managed, and reviewed by authorized providers and staff within a *single health care organization*.

The Health Insurance Portability and Accountability Act (HIPAA) Privacy Rule protects all individually identifiable health information, called *protected health information (PHI)*. PHI includes any electronic, paper, or oral information about health status, the provision of health care, or payment of health care that can be linked to an individual patient.

Within the context of this study guide, the terms EMR and PHI are used. Remember, EMR just refers to records that are used within a health care organization. The term PHI is used when discussing patient's confidential information, which includes clinical records and insurance details.

Privacy Rule. A HIPAA rule that establishes protections for the privacy of individual's health information.

individually identifiable health information. Documents or bits of information that identify the person or provide enough information so that the person could be identified.

How can information be organized within patient charts so that information is easy to find?

ANSWER: One approach is to put similar topics together. For example, all clinical notes should be in one section, and lab reports in another.

FINANCIAL PROCEDURES

An important part of the medical administrative assistant's job is helping manage the office's finances. These tasks involve collecting payments from patients based on their insurance coverage and working with the general bookkeeping system. This section covers both sets of responsibilities.

bookkeeping. Part of the office's accounting functions, to include recording, classifying, and summarizing financial transactions.

Basic Information About Health Insurance

Before the provider sees a patient, the medical administrative assistant must verify the insurance coverage. If a *copayment* is required, many offices prefer to collect it at sign-in.

After each visit, the patient needs a receipt. You may offer a computerized receipt or hand-write one on the spot. Some clinics wait until the end of the visit and issue a copy of the superbill or *encounter form* that includes all charges and payments on the patient's copy.

Most insurance plans have a *deductible*, which is the amount the patient must pay before the insurance pays any charges other than an office visit. Deductibles also vary, often from about $500 to $2,000. Insurance plans usually have deductibles for individuals and for families.

Another feature of insurance plans is *coinsurance*. Coinsurance is a form of cost-sharing that kicks in after the deductible has been met. A typical balance is 80% paid by the insurance company and 20% by the patient.

copayment. A fixed fee for a service or medication, usually collected at the time of service or purchase.

encounter form. A document used to collect data about elements of a patient visit that can become part of a patient record or be used for management purposes.

deductible. The amount a patient must pay before insurance pays anything.

coinsurance. A form of cost-sharing that kicks in after the deductible has been met.

To keep all these variables straight, follow the steps listed below to determine the amount the patient owes and the amount insurance will pay. The end result will be a statement reflecting these charges and reimbursement amounts.

1. Write down the total charge from the explanation of benefits (EOB), which comes from the insurance company, or from the patient's accounts receivable ledger, which is a record of the patients' fees.

2. Subtract the allowable amount from the total charge. The allowable amount is the amount of money you are allowed to collect in most cases. Record the difference either in the adjustments or patient balance column. For example, if the provider writes off the difference as a courtesy, hardship adjustment, or as part of the contract the provider has with the insurance company, the amount is recorded in the adjustments column. If the patient is responsible for paying the difference between the actual charge and the allowable amount, the amount is recorded in the patient balance column.

3. Subtract the deductible amount from the allowable amount. If the deductible is larger than the total amount, subtract only the amount of the deductible that equals the total charge. Then stop. Do not continue with the other steps. Follow the other steps only after the patient's deductible has been met.

4. Identify the coinsurance amount the patient must pay. Let's use 20% as an example. Multiply the total allowable amount by 0.2. Then subtract this coinsurance amount from the total allowed amount balance.

5. Record the deductible and coinsurance amount on separate lines of the patient balance due column of the accounts receivable ledger. That amount is the patient's responsibility. If the patient has secondary insurance, it might be possible to submit the claim to that carrier.

---

statement. A request for payment.

---

explanation of benefits (EOB). A record of a patient's fees.

---

accounts receivable ledger. Document that provides detailed information about charges, payments, and remaining amounts owed to a provider.

Fee Schedules

A provider's fee is based on three variables: time, expertise, and services. Each medical practice and facility is different, so the provider must base fees on these issues as well. Providers generally set the fees for procedures and services. This model is called *fee-for-service.*

As mentioned earlier, third-party payers such as Medicare have influenced what providers can charge by establishing what is called an *allowable charge or allowable amount.* This represents the maximum that the insurance carrier will pay.

---

fee-for-service. Model in which providers set the fees for procedures and services.

---

allowable amount. The limit that most insurance plans put on the amount that will be allowed for reimbursement for a service or procedure.

A change in fee schedules (allowable reimbursement amounts) occurred because of implementation of a *resource-based relative value scale (RBRVS)*. Originally developed for Medicare Part B in 1992, the system now has more widespread use.

According to the RBRVS, fee schedules are created by adding together the following.

- The provider's work

- Charge-based professional liability expenses

- Charge-based overhead

This total is multiplied by a conversion factor, which is a single national number applied to all services paid under the fee schedule.

resource-based relative value scale (RBRVS). System that provides national uniform payments after adjustments across all practices throughout the country.

Medicare Part B. Voluntary supplemental medical insurance to help pay for physicians' and other medical professionals' services, medical services, and medical-surgical supplies not covered by Medicare Part A.

CALCULATING RBRVS

(Physician Work + Malpractice Expense + Practice Expense) ✕ Conversion Factor = Fee Schedule

---

The purpose of the RBRVS system is to provide national uniform payments after adjustments across all practices throughout the country. Conversion factors are changed yearly by Congress and at the request of CMS.

If there is a difference between the provider's fees and what insurance will cover, the provider may be required to write off the difference or pass on the difference to the guarantor, who is responsible for payment.

guarantor. Person or entity responsible for the remaining payment of services after insurance has paid.

Because contracts between providers and insurance carriers vary considerably, it is critical for the medical administrative assistant to know the terms of the contract. When payments are received, the medical administrative assistant must look closely at the EOB from the insurance carrier to make sure that all benefits have been reimbursed correctly.

What factors have helped determine the cost of health care in the past 20 years?

ANSWER: When third-party payers set an allowable amount, they are telling providers that they will only reimburse them up to a certain amount. If providers charge more than that amount, they can try to pass it on to the guarantor, or they may write it off. The RBRVS also imposes limits on provider reimbursement rates and how a patient's coinsurance is charged.

Basic Bookkeeping Information

Along with understanding insurance information, the medical administrative assistant also must be familiar with bookkeeping. *Bookkeeping* is part of the office's accounting functions, which include recording, classifying, and summarizing financial transactions. Recording is the bookkeeper's role in the accounting process.

Bookkeeping must be done every day. In a small practice, the medical administrative assistant might perform these tasks. In a larger practice, these can fall to the office manager or the financial manager.

When performing bookkeeping tasks, follow these guidelines.

- If writing out by hand, use good penmanship so that the records are neat and easy-to-read. Use the same pen style and color of ink consistently. Do not erase, write over, or blot out figures. If an error is made, draw a straight line through the incorrect figure and write the correct figure above it.

- Keep columns of figures straight and clearly formed. It's easy to confuse a "9" and a "7," so make sure the numbers are written clearly.

- Enter all charges and receipts into the daily record or journal as soon as possible. Write a receipt in duplicate for any cash received. Although writing receipts for checks is optional, it's a good idea to have receipts for checks recorded. Post all charges and receipts to the patient ledger every day.

- Checks should be endorsed for deposit as soon as they are received.

- For all other expenses, pay with a check and make sure you have a cancelled check for each payment. Cancelled checks are the best proof of payment. Bills should be paid promptly, before the due date, after they have been reviewed for accuracy. Place the date of payment and the check number on paid bills.

Also, have a *petty cash fund* in place for small, unpredictable expenses, such as postage, parking fees, small contributions, emergency supplies, and miscellaneous small items. In an average-sized facility, $25 to $50 is enough to have on hand. Often, the money is kept in a cashbox or locked drawer. Only one person should be in charge of the petty cash fund. The petty cash fund must be tracked carefully. Every time money is withdrawn, prepare a petty cash voucher for the amount. Then write down each voucher in the petty cash record and enter the new balance. When necessary, add money to the fund. The total of the vouchers plus the fund balance must always equal the beginning amount. Then total the expense columns and post the appropriate accounts in the *disbursement record*. This is the record of the funds distributed to specific expense accounts. Record the amount added to the fund, as well as the new balance in the petty cash fund.

petty cash fund. A small amount of cash available for expenses such as postage, parking fees, small contributions, emergency supplies, and miscellaneous small items.

disbursement. The record of the funds distributed to specific expense accounts.

Kinds of Financial Records

Most offices have two kinds of records: a daily journal and a day sheet. The *daily journal* is a chronological record of bills received, bills paid, and payments and reimbursements received.

The *day sheet* is a daily record of financial transactions. Practices with a pegboard system tend to use day sheets. They include services rendered, charges, and receipts. Every transaction must be recorded on the day sheet to show that the accounts have balanced for the day.

The day sheet is an important reference for preparation of the *end-of-day summary*. This summary has three parts.

- The first part is the proof of posting sections. It refers to the transactions that occurred that day and recorded on the day sheet.

- The second section is the month-to-date accounts receivable proof, which adds the day's totals to the totals already listed.

- The last section is the year-to-date accounts receivable proof, which adds the day's totals to the year-to-date total.

The totals at the bottom of the second and third sections must match. If they do not balance, the medical administrative assistant must check the addition of each column, both vertically and horizontally, to see if there are any computation errors. To avoid mistakes, it is a good idea to use a calculator.

> *daily journal.* A chronological record of bills received, bills paid, and payments and reimbursements received.
>
> *day sheet.* A daily record of financial transactions and services rendered.
>
> *end-of-day summary.* Document consisting of proof of posting sections, month-to-date accounts receivable proof, and year-to-date accounts receivable proof.

Accounting Systems

Two systems are generally used. The *single-entry system* is very basic and mostly used in small offices. It is inexpensive, easy to use, and requires little training.

To implement the single-entry system, three kinds of records are needed.

- The *general journal* is similar to a day sheet, where transactions are entered.

- The *cash payment journal* is a checkbook that is used to make payments.

- The *accounts receivable ledger* provides information about the amounts owed to the provider.

Double-entry bookkeeping is a little more involved and must be done by a trained, experienced bookkeeper or an accountant. In addition to the records needed for a single-entry system, many *subsidiary journals* are needed as well.

The double-entry system is based on the following equation.

> Assets = Liabilities + Proprietorship (Capital)

> *single-entry system.* A method of bookkeeping that relies on a one-sided accounting entry to maintain financial information.
>
> *general journal.* Document where transactions are entered.
>
> *double-entry bookkeeping.* A system in which every entry to an account requires an opposite entry to a different account.
>
> *subsidiary journals.* A document where transactions are summarized and later recorded in a general ledger.

Every transaction must be entered on each side of the accounting equation, and the two sides must always be in balance. *Assets* refer to the properties owned by a business. These include bank accounts, accounts receivable, buildings, equipment, and furniture. The rights to these assets are called *equities*.

The equity of the owner is called capital, proprietorship, or owner's equity. The equity of those to whom money is owed (creditors) are called *liabilities*. The owner's equity or capital is what's left of the assets after the creditors' liabilities have been subtracted.

assets. The properties owned by a business.

equities. What is left of assets after creditors' liabilities have been subtracted.

liabilities. The equity of those to whom money is owed (creditors).

For example, if the provider purchased equipment for $1,000 and put down $250, the provider still owes $750. The equation would look like this:

Assets ($1,000) = Liabilities ($750) + Capital ($250)

The liabilities represent what is still owed, and the capital represents what's been paid. The assets refer to the equipment purchased.

Medical administrative assistants are not trained to manage a double-entry system. Their role is usually just to keep the day journal. For a large practice, the double-entry system is more effective. It provides a more comprehensive financial picture than does the single-entry system.

Invoices and Statements

If an item is not paid when it is purchased, the vendor usually includes an *invoice*. An invoice describes the items and shows the amount due. Invoices should be placed in a designated folder until paid. Some vendors want to be paid based on the invoice.

invoice. A document that describes items purchased or services rendered and shows the amount due.

statement. A request for payment.

Other vendors send a *statement*. A statement is a request for payment. When a patient owes money, the statements are processed monthly. The CMAA often also covers the position of accounts receivable.

Some types of provider offices issue pre-invoices, or quotes. Elective or very expensive procedures can have a pre-invoice issued when insurance will not pay. The patient can look over the quote and secure the funds using the invoice to show a lender.

What is the petty cash fund?

ANSWER: The petty cash fund is a small amount of cash (often $25 to $50) available for expenses such as postage, parking fees, small contributions, emergency supplies, and miscellaneous small items. The money can be kept in a cashbox or locked drawer. Only one person should be in charge of the petty cash fund.

MAIL DELIVERIES

In most offices, a great deal of mail comes in each day. Much of that mail is sent through the U.S. Postal Service (USPS), an independent agency of the executive branch of the U.S. government. USPS provides mail service to every home and business in the United States.

The mail that is sent to medical practices includes the following.

- General correspondence
- Payments for service
- Bills for office purchases
- Insurance claim forms

- Laboratory reports
- Hospital reports
- Medical society mailings
- Professional journals

- Promotional literature
- Advertisements

Every office must establish procedures for defining who is responsible for opening the mail; in what order the letters should be opened; and what pieces, if any, the provider wants to handle. If you are not sure if you should open a piece of mail, do not open it. Rather, send it to the person to whom it is addressed.

Steps for Sorting and Distributing Mail

The following steps are one approach to handling mail in the office.

1. Clear a working space on the desk or countertop for sorting mail.

2. Sort the mail in order of importance.

    a. Provider's personal mail

    b. Ordinary first-class mail

    c. Checks from insurance companies and patients

    d. Periodicals and newspapers

    e. All other pieces

3. Open the mail neatly and in an organized fashion.

4. Stack the envelopes so that they all face the same direction.

5. Pick up the top one and tap the envelope so that when you open it, you won't cut the contents.

6. Open all envelopes along the top edge for easy removal of the contents.

7. Remove the contents of the envelope. Then hold the envelope to the light to make sure there is nothing left inside.

8. When necessary, make a note of the postmark.

9. Discard the envelope after you have made sure that the information inside includes a return address. Some offices prefer to attach the envelope to the correspondence until the mail has been seen.

10. Stamp the letter and any enclosures with the date.

11. If the letter indicates that it is supposed to include an enclosure, make sure it's there. If it isn't, write the word "no" on the letter and circle it.

12. Organize the mail for distribution. Then give each piece of mail to the right person.

Classes of Mail

Mail is classified by type, weight, and destination. Below are the most common types of mail delivered through the USPS.

- *First-class mail:* This is sealed or unsealed typed or handwritten material, including letters, postal cards, postcards, and business reply mail. Postage for mail weighing 13 ounces or less changes frequently. Forever stamps, which are always valid regardless of postal increases, are an efficient way to send first-class mail.

- *Priority mail:* This is first-class mail weighing more than 13 ounces. The postage is calculated based on destination and weight. Priority mail drop shipment is a good way to get mail delivered sooner. Sacks of standard mail are sent to the post office nearest the ZIP code and then sent by standard mail.

- *Standard mail:* This includes advertising, promotional, directory, or editorial material, or any combination of such material. It must be securely bound by permanent fasteners, such as staples or spiral binding. Mail in this class cannot weigh more than 15 pounds.

first-class mail. Sealed or unsealed typed or handwritten material, including letters, postal cards, postcards, and business reply mail.

priority mail. First-class mail weighing more than 13 ounces.

standard mail. Mail that includes advertising, promotional, directory, or editorial material, or any combination of such material.

Special Services

The USPS also offers special services to ensure that the mail arrives at its destination in a timely fashion. Below are some of these options.

- *Insured mail:* This refers to insurance coverage against loss or damage. It is available for priority and first-class mail.

- *Registered mail:* Mail of all classes can be protected by registering it. The sender makes this determination and requests evidence of its delivery. Registered mail must be sent through the post office, where the sender is given a green form to fill out. When the recipient receives the mail, that individual must sign a form acknowledging that the mail arrived. The sender also receives a mailed or online acknowledgment of receipt. There is an extra fee for sending registered mail.

- *Certified mail:* This is first-class mail that also gives the mail added protection. Types of mail that may be sent certified are contracts, deeds, mortgages, bank books, checks, passports, insurance policies, money orders, and birth certificates. Certified mail also requires an additional fee and a special form.

insured mail. Mail that has insurance coverage against loss or damage.

registered mail. Mail of all classes protected by registering and requesting evidence of its delivery.

certified mail. First-class mail that also gives the mail added protection by offering insurance, tracking, and return receipt options.

Private Carriers

In addition to USPS, private companies can deliver mail faster, either overnight or within 1 or 2 days. FedEx is among the most common of these services, but there are others. These include United Parcel Service (UPS), Emery, Airborne Express, and DHL. Most of these companies have central points where packages can be dropped off and sent. Pickup service is also available.

Packing Slips

The vendor usually includes a *packing slip* with the delivery. The packing slip is a list of the items in the package. It's important to check that the items listed on the packing slip are actually in the package.

packing slip. A list of items in a package.

How should mail be sorted?

ANSWER: Mail should be sorted by order of importance.

SUMMARY

This chapter has described many aspects of office management. Depending on the office, the medical administrative assistant is usually involved to some degree in all these activities. These include knowledge of the office filing systems; a basic understanding of electronic records; familiarity with insurance coverage and how to determine what patients owe; a basic understanding of bookkeeping practices; and familiarity with the office's mail sorting, distribution, and delivery policies.

The next chapter covers a very different topic: compliance with federal regulations. There are several sets that medical administrative assistants must understand. These include HIPAA guidelines, regulations for workplace safety established by the Occupational Safety and Health Administration (OSHA), and guidelines established by CMS.

CHAPTER DRILL QUESTIONS

Filing Medical Records

1. What are three filing systems used for paper files?

2. True or False: Cross-reference sheets are needed for numeric filing systems.

3. What is involved in a terminal numbering system?

    a. Giving patients consecutive numbers as they join the practice

    b. Using a combination of a letter and a number

    c. Assigning colors to different numbers.

    d. Assigning consecutive numbers to patients while separating the digits in the number into groups of twos or threes

4. Why is it important to use a good system when filing charts?

Financial Procedures

5. What is the difference between a copayment and coinsurance?

6. True or False: The allowable amount is not taken into account when determining how much the patient owes.

7. What is a day sheet?

8. A provider bought a new piece of equipment for $2,000. The office put down $500 and has a balance of $1,500. What part of the equation is the provider's assets?

    a. The $500 the office put down.

    b. The $1,500 the provider still owes

    c. The $2,000 the provider paid for the new equipment

    d. None of these sums of money are considered assets.

9. What is the difference between an EHR and an EMR?

Mail Deliveries

10. When should registered mail be used?

CHAPTER DRILL ANSWERS

1. Answer: Three filing systems are alphabetic, numeric, and by subject.

2. Answer: True. Because the patient is not identified by name, a cross-reference sheet is needed to match the name with the number.

3. **A.** INCORRECT: This type of system is called consecutive numbering.

   B. INCORRECT: This is an example of a subject filing system.

   C. INCORRECT: This is an example of numeric color-coding.

   D. CORRECT: A terminal numeric system means assigning consecutive patients numbers with the addition of clustering numbers into groups of twos or threes.

4. Answer: The filing system needs to be efficient so that the files are easy to find.

5. Answer: The copayment is a fee collected at the time of service. Coinsurance is the percentage of the health care costs the patient is responsible for after the deductible has been met. Coinsurance may be divided as an 80/20 split, with the insurance carrier paying 80%.

6. Answer: False. The allowable amount is addressed by either having the provider write it off or billing the patient for the difference between the provider's fee and what amount he or she is allowed to charge.

7. Answer: The day sheet is a daily record of financial transactions, including services rendered, charges, and receipts. Every transaction must be recorded on the day sheet to show that the accounts have balanced for the day.

8. **A.** INCORRECT: The $500 is considered to be the provider's capital.

   B. INCORRECT: The $1,500 is considered the provider's liability.

   C. CORRECT: The $2,000 and the equipment it purchased are considered the provider's assets.

   D. INCORRECT: The equipment, at $2,000, is considered the asset.

9. Answer: Registered mail should be used for an important piece of mail that you want to make sure arrives to the recipient. For this reason, the recipient must sign a form indicating that she received the mail. The sender then gets a postcard or digital receipt from USPS stating that the mail arrived at its destination.

10. Answer: The EHR is an electronic record of health-related information about a patient that conforms to nationally recognized interoperability standards that can be created, managed, and reviewed by authorized providers and staff from more than one health care organization. The EMR is an electronic record of health information that is created, added to, managed, and reviewed by authorized providers and staff within a single health care organization.

CHAPTER 4
Compliance

OVERVIEW

In Chapters 2 and 3, the issue of privacy was mentioned in a couple contexts: how the medical staff obtains information from the patient, and when building the patient's health record. In both instances, privacy must be protected at all times, and all medical information must be kept confidential.

This chapter explains in more detail the federal regulations ensuring privacy. In addition, the chapter explains laws enforced by the Occupational Safety and Health Administration (OSHA). These laws are designed to keep the workplace safe. Finally, the chapter presents the basics of preparing paperwork for Medicare and Medicaid claims to prevent fraud.

By the end of this chapter, you should be able to answer the following questions.

1. How does HIPAA protect patients?
2. True or False: When storing files, the minimum necessary is to keep the files turned to the wall so that they cannot be seen by those walking by.
3. What is a Notice of Privacy Practices?
4. With whom are covered entities allowed to share information?
5. When is a patient's privacy not protected?
6. What is an incidental disclosure?
7. What is OSHA's mission?
8. What are the consequences of fraud?
9. What is the difference between Medicare and Medicaid?
10. What are three things that must be in an emergency preparedness plan?

HIPAA GUIDELINES

The Health Insurance Portability and Accountability Act (HIPAA) was enacted in 1996. All health care facilities, insurance companies, and other *covered entities* had to be in compliance by April 14, 2003. The purpose of the law was to create national standards to protect patients' medical records and other personal health information (PHI). Specifically, HIPAA protects patients and providers by:

• Giving patients more control over their medical records.

• Authorizing patients to make informed choices about the uses of their PHI.

• Setting boundaries on the use and release of health records.

• Establishing safeguards that covered entities must follow to ensure that the privacy of health information is protected.

• Holding violators accountable through both civil and criminal penalties if patients' privacy is compromised.

• Protecting the balance struck between public health concerns and the disclosure of PHI.

covered entities. Providers, hospitals, laboratories facilities, nursing homes, rehabilitation facilities, health plans, health care clearinghouses, and those that supply care, services, or supplies to a patient and transmit any health information electronically.

Securing Charts

Chapter 3 discussed how to build files and organize them for easy access. Equally important is placing them in a safe place where patient names cannot be seen. Many providers' offices keep paper files inside a wall folder outside the examination room. If the files are turned so the name is facing the wall, people passing by cannot see the names. This is considered the minimum necessary requirement to protect patient privacy. The hallway should be supervised, and employees should be escorted through this corridor when moving in and out of the office's clinical area.

Using a HIPAA-Compliant Sign-In Sheet

According to HIPAA, patients' names may be called out when it is their turn to see the provider. The office is also allowed to use sign-in sheets. Ideally, most of these sheets allow only one patient to sign in at a time. That way, patients can't see who else is seeing the provider.

For example, some sign-in sheets use pressure-sensitive stickers, which can be removed and placed in the patient's medical record or on a log sheet. Some offices use a computer sign-in system that have the first name of each patient listed on a computer screen about 15 minutes before they are expected to arrive. The patient is told to press "Enter," indicating that he or she has arrived. If the name is not on the screen, the patient is told to see the office staff.

Accessing PHI

Many safeguards are in place to protect patients' confidential information. Although the information in the PHI is about specific patients, the record actually belongs to the provider. The Privacy Rule provides that an individual has a right to adequate notice of how a covered entity may use and disclose protected health information about the individual. For this reason, the patient must be shown the *Notice of Privacy Practices* so that there is no misunderstanding of when and how the PHI can be used.

The Notice of Privacy Practices must include:

- How PHI is used and disclosed by the facility.
- The duties of the provider in protecting health information.
- The patients' rights regarding PHI.
- How complaints can be filed if patients believe their privacy has been violated.
- Whom to contact at the facility for more information.
- The effective date of the Notice of Privacy Practices.

After reading this document, the patient is asked to sign it, which acknowledges that the patient understands the privacy rules. Most patients sign the Notice of Privacy Practices; if, for some reason, the patient refuses, a note to that effect should be placed in the medical record. This proves due diligence on the part of the office and that a good faith effort was made to get the necessary documentation.

After patients sign the Notice of Privacy Practices, providers are allowed to release information to all *covered entities*. Covered entities include health plans, health care clearinghouses that process health information, and providers that transmit information electronically.

Non-covered entities do not have to comply with the Privacy Rule. These include organizations that use, collect, access, and disclose individually identifiable health information. In addition, the Privacy Rule does not apply to all researchers, although some may be considered covered entities. If the researcher is not a covered entity, that individual might have to provide supporting documentation that meets the requirements, conditions, and limitations of the Privacy Rule.

non-covered entities. Organizations that use, collect, access, and disclose individually identifiable health information, but do not transmit electronic data. These do not have to comply with the Privacy Rule.

FIGURE 4.1 *Notice of privacy practices*

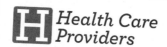

Health Care Providers

1234 Main Street
Shermer, IL 12345
1.800.555.1234

Your Rights

When it c... ...ation, you have certain rights.
...e of our responsibilities to help you.

...opy of your medical record and other health ...his.

...th information, usually within 30 days of your ...e.

... you that you think is incorrect

... why in writing within 60 days.

...example, home or office phone) or to send

...ormation for treatment, payment, or our ...est, and we may say "no" if it would affect

...cket in full, you can ask us not to share that ...ons with your health insurer. We will say "yes"

...shared your health information for six years ...vhy.

...out treatment, payment, and health care ...ou asked us to make). We'll provide one ...cost-based fee if you ask for another one

..., even if you have agreed to receive the ...opy promptly.

...or if someone is your legal guardian, that ...your health information.
...n act for you before we take any action.

...ts by contacting us.
...ealth and Human Services Office for Civil ...S.W., Washington, D.C. 20201, calling ...paa/complaints/.

Health Care Providers

1234 Main Street
Shermer, IL 12345
1.800.555.1234

Notice of Privacy Practices

This notice describes how medical information about you may be used and disclosed and how you can get access to this information.
Please review it carefully.

Overview

Your Rights
You have the right to:
    Get a copy of your paper or electronic medical record
    Correct your paper or electronic medical record
    Request confidential communication
    Ask us to limit the information we share
    Get a list of those with whom we've shared your information
    Get a copy of this privacy notice
    Choose someone to act for you
    File a complaint if you believe your privacy rights have been violated

Your Choices
You have some choices in the way that we use and share information as we:
    Tell family and friends about your condition
    Provide disaster relief
    Include you in a hospital directory
    Provide mental health care
    Market our services and sell your information
    Raise funds

Our Uses and Disclosures
We may use and share your information as we:
    Treat you
    Run our organization
    Bill for your services
    Help with public health and safety issues
    Do research
    Comply with the law
    Respond to organ and tissue donation requests
    Work with a medical examiner or funeral director
    Address workers' compensation, law enforcement, and other government requests
    Respond to lawsuits and legal actions

How Patients Can Access Their Information

Most providers require that patients request access to their PHI in writing and to act on their request within 30 days. Most offices have a form that they use, like the one shown below.

In turn, patients can request restrictions on how their PHI is used. For example, if a patient had an abortion many years ago, she can ask that this information not be released, or *divulged*. The provider does not have to agree to the request, but he must review it and give justification why the restriction cannot be honored. An appeal process should be in place for instances when the provider does not grant the restriction. HIPAA also restricts access to psychotherapy notes, information gathered for legal proceedings, and information exempted from disclosure by the Clinical Laboratory Improvement Amendment (CLIA).

FIGURE 4.2 *Request to access medical record*

Health Care Providers

1234 Main Street
Shermer, IL 12345
1.800.555.1234

Request to Access Medical Record

Patients have the right to access their personal health information. We will be happy to accommodate any patient who wishes to exercise this access to inspect or obtain a copy of the record. Please provide the information requested on this form. This request will be acted upon within thirty (30) days. Standard copy charges will apply.

Print Patient's Name	Date of Birth	Phone

Address	City/State	Zip

Email address	Date of Last Office Visit

Please note below what information should be copied or provided.

Please note below any changes that need to be addressed.

Patient's Signature	Date

Releasing PHI

After the patient signs the Notice of Privacy Practices document, the provider may disclose information as authorized by the document. Virtually all treatment, payment, and operations (TPO) are covered under the privacy practices document.

Some offices provide a receipt after patients have signed the privacy practices document. Others post the document prominently in the office. No matter which approach the office uses, there must be a signed copy in every patient's medical record.

HIPAA regulations allow medical staff to send a fax containing PHI to another provider for treatment purposes or to another individual as requested by the patient. When sending a fax, make sure to verify the numbers, direct the fax to a certain person, and use cover sheets that stress confidentiality. All fax machines should be located in secure areas to prevent unauthorized access to PHI. Information can also be shared with other providers by phone or email, as long as precautions are taken.

Sometimes conflicts arise as to how much information to release. For example, a patient signs a release requesting that all his medical information be sent to his attorney. But then, the attorney forwards a signed release requesting just progress notes. In a situation like this, call the patient first and attempt to verify the request. Alternatively, the office could choose to adhere to the more restrictive request. Always document any form of communication about patient preferences in writing. In some cases, the patient needs to sign a new permission form. It's always better to contact the patient and ask for clarification than to divulge too much information.

> *divulge.* Make private or sensitive information known.

Sharing Information with Family and Friends

According to the Privacy Rule, covered entities are allowed to share information relevant to the patient's care with a spouse, family members, friends, or other individuals identified by the patient. The covered entity is also allowed to share relevant information if it can reasonably be inferred, based on professional judgment, that the patient does not object or that the action is in the patient's best interest. But if the patient has requested that such information not be shared, then the provider must honor that request unless she considers it unreasonable. Then, this must be documented.

If the patient has authorized that information can be shared, it is up to providers to develop a system to verify the identity of the person receiving the information. For example, the medical administrative assistant can ask to see a driver's license to make sure the information is being given to the right person.

For billing purposes, both covered entities and *business associates* can discuss issues related to reimbursement with some people other than the patient. There is also a limit on the amount of information that can be shared. Such disclosures must be in accordance with the minimum necessary standard, which states that "protected health information should not be used or disclosed when it is not necessary to satisfy a particular purpose or carry out a function." Providers also must abide by reasonable requests by the patient for confidential communications and restrictions.

> *business associates.* Individuals, groups, or organizations, who are not members of a covered entity's workforce, that perform functions or activities on behalf of or for a covered entity.

If the patient is a child, parents are allowed to see medical records as long as this practice is consistent with state law. In fact, parents are usually the child's personal representatives under the Privacy Rule.

In some cases, however, the parent is not considered the child's personal representative. These cases include the following.

- When the minor is the one who consents to care and the parent's consent is not required under state or any other law

- When the minor obtains care at the direction of a court or a person appointed by the court

- When the parent agrees that the minor and the provider might have a confidential relationship

When Privacy Is Not Protected

When public health concerns are involved, an individual's PHI is not protected under the Privacy Rule. These include:

- Access to records from a nursing home to ensure that the providers are caring for the residents properly and the facility is clean.

- Protecting the public from epidemics, such as reporting a flu epidemic in a particular area, cases of sexually transmitted diseases (STDs), or cases of HIV/AIDS.

- Making required reports to police, such as reporting a gunshot wound, or to child protective services, if there are concerns about abuse.

Communicating With Patients

In the provider's office, sometimes it's impossible for patients to avoid seeing a name on a sign-in sheet or hearing a patient's name being called out. This kind of information, which other people can see or hear, is referred to as an *incidental disclosure*. An incidental disclosure is a secondary use that cannot be reasonably prevented, is limited in nature, and occurs as a result of another use or disclosure that is permitted. These kinds of disclosures are permitted under HIPAA.

Other examples of incidental disclosures include:

- Confidential conversations between providers or with patients, if there is a possibility that they may be overheard (e.g., by hearing the patient and provider talking through the wall when in an adjacent examining room).

- Seeing other patients when signing in.

- A person not authorized to see PHI walking by medical equipment and seeing material containing *individually identifiable health information*, such as a person's name on an ultrasound screen.

- Health care staff coordinating patient care services at a nurses' station or central location in an office.

- A pharmacist discussing a patient with a provider on the phone when another person is standing nearby.

---

incidental disclosure. Secondary use of PHI that cannot be reasonably prevented, is limited in nature, and occurs as a result of another use or disclosure that is permitted.

Sometimes medical administrative assistants must communicate with patients outside the office. Usually the first attempt is by phone. If the patient doesn't answer, then it's up to the medical administrative assistant to decide whether to leave a message and how much information to disclose if someone else picks up. Even leaving a message on an answering machine can be questionable because there is no way to know who can hear that message. Have patients list acceptable methods of contact and leaving messages when they complete their intake forms.

Patients have the option of requesting that they be contacted in a confidential manner. For example, patients may ask to be contacted at work instead of at home.

What are three ways that HIPAA guidelines benefit the patient?

> **ANSWER:** HIPAA guidelines benefit patients by giving them more control of their medical records; authorizing them to be able to make informed choices about the uses of their PHI; and setting boundaries on the use and release of health records.

Electronic PHI

As electronic record-keeping increases in medical practices, it is important to ensure the confidentiality of PHI in that format. One part of HIPAA, called *HIPAA Administrative Simplification,* focuses on protecting electronic information. It does so by requiring the use of standardized electronic formats when sending administrative and financial data.

The electronic transmission of data is called *electronic data interchange (EDI)*. It refers to the exchange of routine business transactions from one computer to another using publicly available communications protocols. In medical practices, standardized EDI formats are required. These standards, recently revised to accommodate ICD-10-CM, is called ASC X12 Version 5010 standards.

electronic data interchange (EDI). The transfer of electronic information in a standard format.

HIPAA standards cover electronic transactions frequently made between medical offices and health plans. Such exchanges contain forms with sensitive information. For this reason, medical practices must use specific electronic formats for each kind of transaction. These are listed in Table 4.1.

TABLE 4.1 *Required electronic formats*

TYPE OF FORMAT	USE
X12 270/271: Health Care Eligibility Benefit Inquiry and Response	Questions and answers on whether patients' health plans cover planned treatments and procedures.
X12 276/277: Health Care Claim Status Request and Response	Questions and answers between providers, such as medical offices and hospitals, and payers about claims that are due to be paid.
X12 278: Health Care Services Review—Request for Review and Response	Questions and answers between patients, or providers on their behalf, and managed care organizations for approval to see medical specialists.
X12 835: Claims Payment and Remittance Advice (RA)	The payment and RA are sent from the payer to the provider. The payment may be sent electronically from the payer directly to the provider's bank.
X12 837: Health Care Claim or Encounter	Data about the billing provider who requests payment, the patient, the diagnoses, and the procedures sent by a provider to a payer.

The *X12 837 Health Claim Form,* or 837P for short, is referred to as the professional claim because it is used to bill for a provider's services. Practices must use other formats for hospital claims, or institutional claims, and still other formats for drug claims.

National Provider Identifier (NPI). Unique 10-digit code for providers required by HIPAA.

Another HIPAA requirement is the use of a *national standard identifier* for all providers. The *National Provider Identifier (NPI)* is a 10-number identifier that keeps any information about the provider (location, specialization) confidential.

HIPAA Security Rule

The HIPAA Security Rule describes safeguards that must be in place to protect the confidentiality, integrity, and availability of health information stored in a computer and transmitted across computer networks, including the Internet.

The security standards are divided into the following three categories.

- *Administrative safeguards*: These are administrative policies and procedures designed to protect electronic health information. One individual in the office should have this responsibility. This person should begin by conducting an assessment of the current level of data security. With that information in hand, security policies and procedures should be developed, followed by annual training to educate staff members about these policies.

- *Physical safeguards*: These include the mechanisms required to protect electronic systems, equipment, and data from threats, environmental hazards, and unauthorized intrusion. Such threats can come from computer hackers, disgruntled employees, and angry patients. Environmental hazards include unplanned system outages or floods. Information can be protected by backing up the computer daily. The backup files should then be stored in a different physical location for safekeeping.

- *Technical safeguards*: These are automated processes to protect and control access to data. Access should only be granted on an as-needed basis. For example, the staff member responsible for scheduling does not need access to billing information. Ensuring that usernames and passwords are kept confidential is another technical safeguard. Others include antivirus and firewall software and secure transmission systems for sending patient data from one computer to another.

An additional security measure is an *audit trail*, which is a report that traces who has accessed electronic information, when the information was accessed, and whether any information was changed. The person in charge of security should review the report regularly for irregularities.

HIPAA Security Rule. Rule that describes safeguards that must be in place to protect the confidentiality, integrity, and availability of health information stored in a computer and transmitted across computer networks, including the Internet.

firewall. Part of a computer system that blocks unauthorized access while allowing outward communication.

audit trail. A report that traces who has accessed electronic information.

Peer-to-Peer Information

Peer-to-peer file-sharing software allows computers to download files and make them available to other people on the network. Such software presents potential security risks. To make sure health information remains secure, the Health Information Technology for Economic and Clinical Health (HITECH) Act sets requirements for increased protection. This added security is provided by using technologies that makes the PHI "unusable, unreadable, or undecipherable to unauthorized individuals." If a breach occurs, providers, health plans, and other covered entities are required to notify patients, the federal government, and the media.

To provide quality care for patients, providers can exchange clinical information with other providers in different locations through the use of local, state, and regional health information network. A *health information exchange (HIE)* enables the sharing of health-related information among providers according to nationally recognized standards.

> *health information exchange (HIE).* System that enables the sharing of health-related information among providers according to nationally recognized standards.

How does HIPAA ensure the confidentiality of electronic PHI?

ANSWER: HIPAA ensures the confidentiality of electronic PHI through administrative, physical, and technical safeguards.

Penalties for Violating HIPAA Practices

The medical staff must be aware of the penalties involved for not following HIPAA regulations. Individuals can be held liable for neglecting to follow the regulations. Table 4.2 outlines types of HIPAA violations, as well as the minimum and maximum penalties. These penalties are fall under civil law. In some instances, covered entities may also face criminal penalties, which involve time in prison. Knowingly obtaining or disclosing PHI, offenses committed under false pretenses, and offenses committed with the intent of selling, using, or transferring PHI are examples of offenses that are considered to be criminal.

TABLE 4.2 *HIPAA violations and penalties*

HIPAA VIOLATION	MINIMUM PENALTY	MAXIMUM PENALTY
Individual did not know (and by exercising reasonable diligence would not have known) that he violated HIPAA	$100 per violation, with an annual maximum of $25,000 for repeat violations (maximum that can be imposed by State Attorneys General regardless of the type of violation)	$50,000 per violation, with an annual maximum of $1.5 million
HIPAA violation due to reasonable cause and not due to willful neglect	$1,000 per violation, with an annual maximum of $100,000 for repeat violations	$50,000 per violation, with an annual maximum of $1.5 million
HIPAA violation due to willful neglect but violation is corrected within the required time period	$10,000 per violation, with an annual maximum of $250,000 for repeat violations	$50,000 per violation, with an annual maximum of $1.5 million
HIPAA violation is due to willful neglect and is not corrected	$50,000 per violation, with an annual maximum of $1.5 million	$50,000 per violation, with an annual maximum of $1.5 million

Source: AMA, www.ama-assn.org

OSHA GUIDELINES

The Occupational Safety and Health Administration (OSHA) was established in 1970, when President Nixon signed the Occupational Safety and Health Act. Part of the U.S. Department of Labor, its mission is to ensure workplace safety and a healthy working environment. Since its founding, workplace injuries, illnesses, and fatalities have reduced significantly.

Occupational Safety and Health Administration (OSHA). Part of the U.S. Department of Labor with the mission to ensure workplace safety and a healthy working environment.

Originally, OSHA's focus was on construction workers and engineers. But in the late 1980s, when HIV was identified, it became clear that actions were needed to protect medical staff who worked with patients with infectious diseases. OSHA's Final Rule on Bloodborne Pathogens became effective in 1992. Since then, it has been updated in light of new information about these pathogens. This law requires medical facilities to comply with the Bloodborne Pathogens Standard and to be able to prove compliance to OSHA inspectors.

To ensure that other workplace hazards are covered, OSHA's General Duty Clause fits almost any situation not covered in another section of the law. This clause states that every workplace must be free of any hazard that might cause serious harm or death.

Exposure Control Plan

Each facility must have a written *exposure control plan* in place. The plan describes the tasks employees must perform if there is a risk of exposure to blood or other potentially infectious materials, and what procedures are in place to track employee exposures.

The exposure control plan also must have a waste management section that explains how waste is removed from the facility and destroyed. Many medical offices contract with companies that specialize in removing and destroying medical waste. The office must keep these companies' receipts to prove that this material was handled correctly.

Another part of the plan is a section on hazardous materials communication. This section documents what substances in the facility are hazardous and how to handle a spill or exposure to them. The manufacturer of the chemical is the only party that can determine whether it is hazardous. To document this information, material safety data sheets (SDSs) must be kept on almost all chemicals and reagents in the facility. Some chemicals have been exempted from documentation, but without the SDS information, it is difficult to determine what type of health, reactivity, flammability, or other risks the chemical could have. Therefore, keeping SDS records on chemicals is required.

exposure control plan. Plan that describes tasks employees must perform if there is a risk of exposure to blood or other potentially infectious materials, and what procedures are in place to track employee exposures.

Reporting an OSHA Incident

Although medical and dental clinics are exempt from maintaining OSHA 300 Series Injury and Illness logs, it is important to know about the reporting process. An injury or illness is considered work-related when an event or exposure in the workplace contributed to or caused the condition or significantly aggravated a pre-existing condition. To track work-related injuries, OSHA requires that the following records be kept.

- *OSHA Form 300 (Log of Work-Related Injuries and Illnesses):* This form documents work-related deaths and every work-related injury or illness that involves loss of consciousness, restricted work activity or job transfer, days away from work, or medical treatment beyond first aid. *OSHA Form 301 (Injury and Illness Incident Report)* should be completed for each entry in the log.

- *OSHA Form 300A (Summary of Work-Related Injuries and Illnesses):* This form must be completed even if no work-related injuries or illnesses occurred during the year. This information must be posted publicly in the facility for 1 to 3 months, from February 1 to April 30. A company executive must examine the document and certify that it is accurate.

- *OSHA Form 301 (Injury and Illness Incident Report):* This form is used to report what happened when an employee experiences a work-related injury or illness. This form (or an acceptable substitute, such as a state workers' compensation form) must be completed within 7 calendar days after notification of the injury or illness.

In filling out the form, follow these steps.

- Interview the employee or employees involved in the incident.

- Review the notes taken by those who witnessed the incident.

- Interview those who might have additional information or who provided the original notes if clarification is needed.

- Read through OSHA Form 301 before filling it out.

- Complete information about the employee or employees and the health care professional who treated them.

- Describe in detail the information requested about the incident, including the injury or illness, a narrative of what happened, and what objects were involved in the injury.

- Sign the report. If possible, review it with the employee or employees involved.

- If the injured employee or employees completed an incident report, make sure it's reviewed and signed by a supervisor.

- Make sure the incident was reported in a timely manner and within any state regulatory times.

- Refer the employee or employees to the proper individuals for medical care.

The log and summary forms should be kept on file for a minimum of 5 years. Only the summary needs to be posted. These forms are not sent to OSHA unless requested. If you have any phone contact with OSHA, it is a good idea to keep a record of these calls. Be sure to include the name of the person you spoke to, that person's title, questions asked, and responses given. This record could be important if an OSHA inspector comes to the facility or raises questions about safety practices.

Emergency Preparedness

Every medical facility with more than 10 employees must have a written emergency plan in place. The plan must have procedures for the following.

- Reporting fire or other emergency

- Performing an emergency evacuation, including the type of evacuation and exit route assignments

- Establishing rules for employees who remain to run critical equipment before they evacuate

- Accounting for all employees after evacuation

- Establishing procedures to be followed by employees performing rescue or medical duties

- Providing the name or title of the person (or persons) to be contacted about the plan or an explanation of the individual's duties under the plan

In addition, the plan must have an alarm system to notify employees of an emergency, and the system must use a separate, distinct signal for each type of emergency. Employees must be trained in safe evacuation procedures, and the plan must be reviewed with each employee at the following times.

- When the plan is developed

- When the employee is initially assigned to a job

- When the employee's responsibilities change

- When the plan is changed

Facilities with more than 10 employees also must have a written fire prevention plan that includes the following.

- A list of all major fire hazards with the proper handling and storage of each

- The type of fire prevention equipment necessary to control each major hazard

- Procedures to control accumulations of flammable and combustible waste materials

- Procedures for regular maintenance of safeguards installed on heat-producing equipment to prevent the accidental ignition of combustible materials

- The name or job title of the person responsible for maintaining equipment, preventing or controlling sources of ignition or fires, and controlling fuel source hazards

Employees must be told about any fire hazards associated with their job. There also should be procedures in place about natural disasters, such as hurricanes and tornadoes, and criminal incidents, such as robbery or vandalism. Large-scale events, such as terrorist attacks or bioterrorism, also should be addressed because medical professionals can be needed to help in these situations.

Evacuation Plans

Evacuations can only take place after a safety officer has given the order. When leaving the facility, keep the lights on. The exits must be clear so that all patients and employees can get out safely. Then all evacuees should try the first exit route. If it becomes impassible, use the second route.

The people nearest the danger should be evacuated first, followed by an orderly evacuation of the rest of the people in the facility. Close all doors after people have safely left the facility. If moving through smoke-filled areas, keep low and do not run. If doors feel warm or give off smoke when opened slightly, do not go into those rooms.

When all staff and patients are out of the facility, take them to a designated area. Leave one person behind to ensure that no one returns to the facility. Keep a count of all people, and notify the safety officer is anyone is missing.

If required, what form should be used to report an incident to OSHA?

ANSWER: OSHA Form 301 should be used to report an incident.

CENTER FOR MEDICARE/MEDICAID SERVICES (CMS) GUIDELINES

Difference Between Medicare and Medicaid

CMS oversees two important government insurance programs: Medicare and Medicaid. *Medicare* is a federal health insurance program that provides health care coverage for individuals age 65 and older. The program also covers people younger than 65 who have disabilities.

Medicaid provides insurance for people who are considered medically indigent. Under this program, the government works with the states to provide medical care for people who meet specific eligibility criteria.

Medicare and Medicaid Fraud

Special claim forms must be filled out for recipients of Medicare and Medicaid. Strict laws are in place regulating how to complete these forms. If these rules are not followed, individuals are at risk for committing *fraud.*

CMS defines fraud as "making false statements of representations of material facts to obtain some benefit or payment for which no entitlement would otherwise exist." In other words, fraud is when something is said that is not true for the purposes of receiving payments. Billing for a service that was not rendered is an example of fraud.

Specific examples of fraud include the following.

- Knowingly billing for services or supplies not provided, including billing Medicare or Medicaid for appointments that the patient failed to keep.

- Knowingly altering claim forms to receive a higher payment. Upcoding is an example of this.

fraud. Making false statements of representations of material facts to obtain some benefit or payment for which no entitlement would otherwise exist.

Upcoding is when a diagnosis or procedure code is assigned specifically to receive a higher level of payment. Assigning a cough with the code for pneumonia is an example of upcoding.

---

upcoding. Assigning a diagnosis or procedure code at a higher level than the documentation supports, such as coding bronchitis as pneumonia.

---

unbundling. Using multiple codes that describe different components of a treatment instead of using a single code that describes all steps of the procedure.

---

program abuse. Practices that, either directly or indirectly, result in unnecessary costs to government-funded programs.

Another way codes can be misused is through *unbundling.* Unbundling is the practice of using multiple codes that describe different components of a treatment instead of using the correct single code that describes all steps of the procedure

Abuse refers to practices that, either directly or indirectly, result in unnecessary costs to the Medicare program. Abuse includes any practice that is not consistent with the goals of providing patients with services that are medically necessary, meet professionally recognized standards, and are fairly priced.

Other examples of abuse include the following.

- Charging excessively for services or supplies

- Billing for services that were not medically necessary

- Misusing codes on a claim

What is fraud?

ANSWER: CMS defines fraud as making false statements of representations of material facts to obtain some benefit or payment for which no entitlement would otherwise exist. In other words, fraud is when something is said that is not true for the purposes of receiving payments.

Reporting Fraud

In addition to playing a key role in ensuring privacy, HIPAA also has regulations related to fraud and abuse. The key areas targeted by HIPAA are *medical necessity,* or providing appropriate care for a given diagnosis; upcoding; unbundling; and billing for services not provided.

The law also mandated that information about fraud and abuse be compiled into a data bank called the national *Healthcare Integrity and Protection Data Bank (HIPDB).* According to the Department of Health and Human Services (HHS), the types of information that must be reported to HIPDB include the following.

- Federal or state licensing and certification actions, including revocation, reprimands, censures, probations, suspensions, and any other loss of license, or the right to apply for or renew a license, whether by voluntary surrender, non-renewability, or otherwise.

- Exclusion from participation in federal or state health care programs.

- Any other actions or decisions defined in the HIPDB regulations.

---

medical necessity. The documented need for a particular medical intervention.

Healthcare Integrity and Protection Data Bank (HIPDB). A compilation of information about fraud and abuse.

Only federal and state government agencies are required to report such violations. Access to HIPDB is limited to those organizations, as well as practitioners, providers, and suppliers.

Consequences of Fraud

HIPAA established a comprehensive program to combat fraud called the *Health Care Fraud and Abuse Program (HCFAP)*. Housed in the Office of Inspector General (OIG), the program is run jointly by the Department of Justice and HHS. The OIG protects Medicare and other HHS programs from fraud and abuse by conducting audits, investigations, and inspections.

> ***Health Care Fraud and Abuse Program (HCFAP).*** Program that protects Medicare and other HHS programs from fraud and abuse by conducting audits, investigations, and inspections.

The OIG has the authority to exclude individuals and entities who have engaged in fraud and abuse from participating in Medicare, Medicaid, and other federal health care programs. The office also can impose penalties on offenders. The OIG keeps an office List of Excluded Individuals/Entities (LEIE).

In 2009, the Department of Justice and HHS established the *Health Care Fraud Prevention and Enforcement Action Team (HEAT)* to strengthen efforts to fight fraud and invest in new technologies to prevent both fraud and abuse. The website www.stopmedicarefraud.gov provides information about how to identify fraud and report it.

CMS-1500 Form

The Administrative Simplification Compliance Act (ASCA) requires that claims to Medicare be transmitted electronically. But if a provider uses a clearinghouse to submit claims, the draft sent to the clearinghouse may be completed on paper. For paper claims, the correct form to use is CMS-1500, which has been revised by the organization that maintains it, the National Uniform Claim Committee (NUCC). Any new version of the form must be approved by the White House Office of Management and Budget (OMB). OMB has approved the revised form, referred to as version 02/12, OMB control number 0938-1197.

It is very important to fill out the form correctly. The following section explains what information (referred to as blocks) needs to go in each field.

FIGURE 4.3 *CMS-1500*

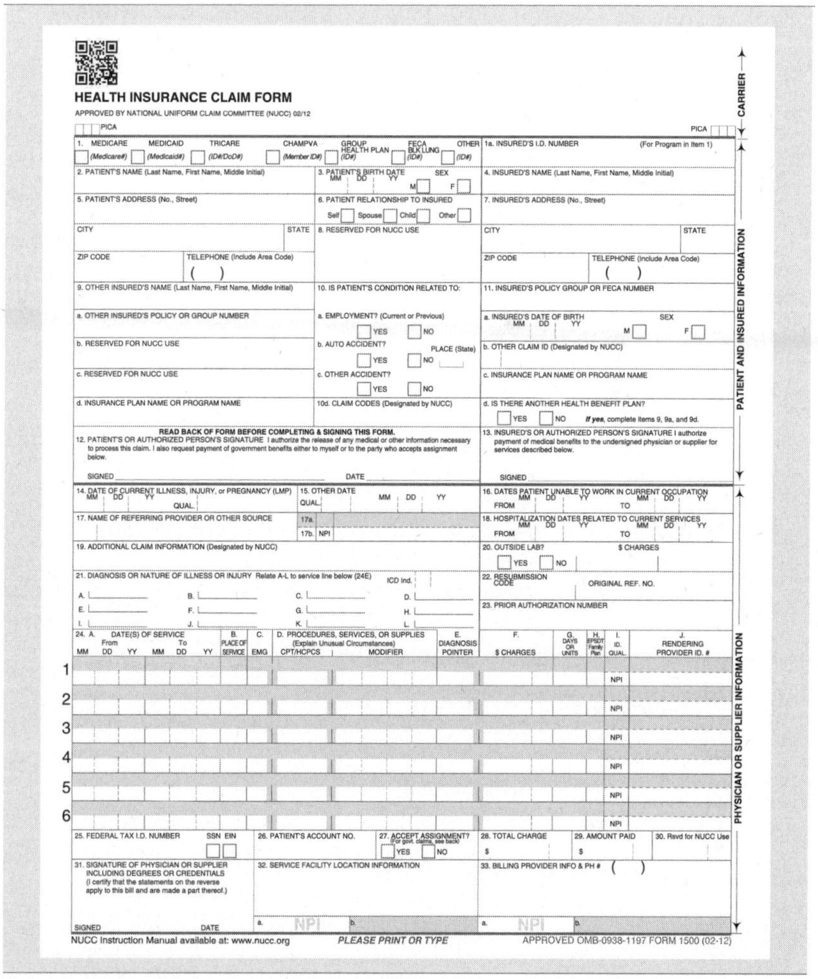

HEALTH INSURANCE CLAIM FORM
APPROVED BY NATIONAL UNIFORM CLAIM COMMITTEE (NUCC) 02/12

PICA | PICA

1. MEDICARE (Medicare#) MEDICAID (Medicaid#) TRICARE (ID#/DoD#) CHAMPVA (Member ID#) GROUP HEALTH PLAN (ID#) FECA BLK LUNG (ID#) OTHER (ID#)
1a. INSURED'S I.D. NUMBER (For Program in Item 1)
2. PATIENT'S NAME (Last Name, First Name, Middle Initial)
3. PATIENT'S BIRTH DATE MM DD YY SEX M F
4. INSURED'S NAME (Last Name, First Name, Middle Initial)
5. PATIENT'S ADDRESS (No., Street)
6. PATIENT RELATIONSHIP TO INSURED Self Spouse Child Other
7. INSURED'S ADDRESS (No., Street)
CITY STATE
8. RESERVED FOR NUCC USE
CITY STATE
ZIP CODE TELEPHONE (Include Area Code) ( )
ZIP CODE TELEPHONE (Include Area Code) ( )
9. OTHER INSURED'S NAME (Last Name, First Name, Middle Initial)
10. IS PATIENT'S CONDITION RELATED TO:
11. INSURED'S POLICY GROUP OR FECA NUMBER
a. OTHER INSURED'S POLICY OR GROUP NUMBER
a. EMPLOYMENT? (Current or Previous) YES NO
a. INSURED'S DATE OF BIRTH MM DD YY SEX M F
b. RESERVED FOR NUCC USE
b. AUTO ACCIDENT? YES NO PLACE (State)
b. OTHER CLAIM ID (Designated by NUCC)
c. RESERVED FOR NUCC USE
c. OTHER ACCIDENT? YES NO
c. INSURANCE PLAN NAME OR PROGRAM NAME
d. INSURANCE PLAN NAME OR PROGRAM NAME
10d. CLAIM CODES (Designated by NUCC)
d. IS THERE ANOTHER HEALTH BENEFIT PLAN? YES NO *If yes*, complete items 9, 9a, and 9d.
READ BACK OF FORM BEFORE COMPLETING & SIGNING THIS FORM.
12. PATIENT'S OR AUTHORIZED PERSON'S SIGNATURE I authorize the release of any medical or other information necessary to process this claim. I also request payment of government benefits either to myself or to the party who accepts assignment below.
SIGNED DATE
13. INSURED'S OR AUTHORIZED PERSON'S SIGNATURE I authorize payment of medical benefits to the undersigned physician or supplier for services described below.
SIGNED
14. DATE OF CURRENT ILLNESS, INJURY, or PREGNANCY (LMP) MM DD YY QUAL.
15. OTHER DATE QUAL. MM DD YY
16. DATES PATIENT UNABLE TO WORK IN CURRENT OCCUPATION FROM MM DD YY TO MM DD YY
17. NAME OF REFERRING PROVIDER OR OTHER SOURCE 17a. 17b. NPI
18. HOSPITALIZATION DATES RELATED TO CURRENT SERVICES FROM MM DD YY TO MM DD YY
19. ADDITIONAL CLAIM INFORMATION (Designated by NUCC)
20. OUTSIDE LAB? YES NO $ CHARGES
21. DIAGNOSIS OR NATURE OF ILLNESS OR INJURY Relate A-L to service line below (24E) ICD Ind.
A. B. C. D. E. F. G. H. I. J. K. L.
22. RESUBMISSION CODE ORIGINAL REF. NO.
23. PRIOR AUTHORIZATION NUMBER
24. A. DATE(S) OF SERVICE From MM DD YY To MM DD YY | B. PLACE OF SERVICE | C. EMG | D. PROCEDURES, SERVICES, OR SUPPLIES (Explain Unusual Circumstances) CPT/HCPCS MODIFIER | E. DIAGNOSIS POINTER | F. $ CHARGES | G. DAYS OR UNITS | H. EPSDT Family Plan | I. ID. QUAL. | J. RENDERING PROVIDER ID. #
1 NPI
2 NPI
3 NPI
4 NPI
5 NPI
6 NPI
25. FEDERAL TAX I.D. NUMBER SSN EIN
26. PATIENT'S ACCOUNT NO.
27. ACCEPT ASSIGNMENT? (For govt. claims, see back) YES NO
28. TOTAL CHARGE $
29. AMOUNT PAID $
30. Rsvd for NUCC Use
31. SIGNATURE OF PHYSICIAN OR SUPPLIER INCLUDING DEGREES OR CREDENTIALS (I certify that the statements on the reverse apply to this bill and are made a part thereof.)
SIGNED DATE
32. SERVICE FACILITY LOCATION INFORMATION a. NPI b.
33. BILLING PROVIDER INFO & PH # ( ) a. NPI b.
NUCC Instruction Manual available at: www.nucc.org PLEASE PRINT OR TYPE APPROVED OMB-0938-1197 FORM 1500 (02-12)

CARRIER | PATIENT AND INSURED INFORMATION | PHYSICIAN OR SUPPLIER INFORMATION

Source: National Uniform Claim Committee

Member Information

Blocks 1 through 13 focus on basic information about the patient, the insured (if that person is different), and determining which plan is primary and which is secondary if the patient has two insurance plans (Block 11). This information must be entered exactly as specified.

FIGURE 4.4 *CMS-1500 Form Blocks 1-8*

Source: National Uniform Claim Committee

BLOCK 1	Check the box indicating what kind of insurance is applicable, such as Medicare.
BLOCK 1A	The patient's *Medicare Health Insurance Claim Number (HICN)*. This number must be recorded whether Medicare is the primary or secondary payer.
BLOCK 2	The patient's first name, middle initial (if any), and last name, as shown on the patient's Medicare card.
BLOCK 3	The patient's eight-digit birth date recorded as MM|DD|CCYY and sex. For example, September 28, 1990, would be recorded 09|28|1990.
BLOCK 4	If there is insurance primary to Medicare, obtained through the patient's or spouse's place of work or through any other source, list the name of the insured here. If the patient and the insured are the same, write SAME. If Medicare is primary, leave this field blank.
BLOCK 5	The patient's mailing address and telephone number. Put the mailing address on the first line, the city and state on the second line, and the ZIP code and phone number on the third line.
BLOCK 6	Check the appropriate box for patient's relationship to the insured.
BLOCK 7	Enter the insured's address and phone number. If the insured is the same as the patient, write SAME. Complete this block only after blocks 4, 6, and 11 have been completed.
BLOCK 8	Leave blank.

FIGURE 4.5 *CMS-1500 Form Blocks 9-13*

Source: National Uniform Claim Committee

BLOCK 9   Write the last name, first name, and middle initial (if there is one) of the Medigap enrollee if it is a different person from the one listed in Block 2. Otherwise, write SAME. If no Medigap benefits are assigned, leave blank.

BLOCK 9A   Enter the policy and/or group number of the Medigap insured preceded by MEDIGAP, MG, or MGAP.

BLOCK 9B   Leave blank.

BLOCK 9C   Leave blank.

BLOCK 9D   Write in the Coordination of Benefits Agreement Medigap-based identifier.

BLOCKS 10A-10C   Check "Yes" or "No" to indicate whether employment, auto liability, or other accident involvement applies to one or more of the services listed in block 24. A "yes" answer indicates there may be other insurance primary to Medicare.

> *Medigap.* A private health insurance that pays for most of the charges not covered by Parts A and B.

BLOCK 11   This is an important field. This is the place to indicate that a good faith effort has been made to determine whether Medicare is the primary insurance. Information about insurance primary to Medicare should be listed in blocks 11a-11c.

Instances where Medicare is the secondary insurance include the following.

- Group health plan coverage
  - Working aged
  - Disability (large group health plan)
  - End-stage renal disease
- No-fault or other liability
- Work-related illness/injury
  - Workers' compensation
  - Black lung
  - Veterans benefits

BLOCK 11A   This is where the insured's birth date goes. Enter the sex as well if it is different from Block 3.

BLOCK 11B   For insurance primary to Medicare, enter employer's name, if applicable. If there is a change in the insured's insurance status (e.g., retired), enter either a 6-digit (MMDDYY) or 8-digit (MMDDCCYY) retirement date preceded by the word "RETIRED." For Tricare and CHAMPVA, enter the sponsor's branch of service, using abbreviations (e.g., United States Navy = USN). For commercial claims, check for payer-specific instructions.

BLOCK 11C   Enter the nine-digit payer ID number of the primary insurer. If there is no payer ID, then write in the primary payer's program or plan name. If the explanation of benefits (EOB) does not include the claim's processing address, then write it in.

BLOCK 11D   For Medicare, leave blank. For all other payers, enter an "x" in the correct box, if appropriate. If marked "YES," complete items 9, 9a, and 9d.

BLOCKS 12   This is an important field. This is the place where the patient or an authorized person signs to authorize the release of medical information. The field must be dated and entered as a six- or eight-digit date. A signature on file or a computer-generated signature can also be used. The patient's signature authorizes release of information necessary to process the claim.

BLOCK 13   This signature authorizes payment of benefits to the provider or supplier. A signature on file is acceptable here.

Why is Block 11 important?

ANSWER: This is the place to indicate that a good faith effort has been made to determine which is the primary insurance and which is secondary.

Provider of Service (POS) or Supplier Information

These fields (14 to 33) include information about the providers, services rendered, diagnoses made, procedures performed, and modifiers needs. Each field is described below.

FIGURE 4.6 *CMS-1500 Form Blocks 14-18*

Source: National Uniform Claim Committee

BLOCK 14   For Medicare, for the current illness, injury, or pregnancy, enter either an 8-digit (MMDDCCYY) or 6-digit (MMDDYY) date. For chiropractic services, enter the date of the initiation of the course of treatment and enter the date of x-ray (if used to demonstrate subluxation) in item 19. Medicare does not use qualifiers.

For commercial claims: Enter the date of the first date of the present illness, injury, or pregnancy. For pregnancy, use the date of the last menstrual period (LMP) as the first date. Enter the applicable qualifier to identify which date is being reported (e.g., 431 Onset of Current Symptoms or Illness, 484 Last Menstrual Period).

BLOCK 15   For Medicare, leave blank (not required). For all other carriers, check for payer-specific instructions. When required, enter another date related to the patient's condition or treatment and the applicable qualifier to identify which date is being reported.

BLOCK 16   Dates patient is unable to work in his/her current occupation. This is required if the patient is eligible for disability or workers' compensation benefits. To fill out this field, enter the "From" and "To" dates as follows: MMDDYY (051512) or MMDDCCYY (05152012).

BLOCK 17   This is where the name of the referring or ordering provider goes. If Medicare requires that a supervising provider be listed, this is where to put that name. If a claim involves more than one referring, ordering, or supervising provider, a separate claim must be submitted for each one. Table 4.3 shows the qualifiers that should be used for each kind of provider.

TABLE 4.3 *Qualifiers for different kinds of providers*

QUALIFIER	PROVIDER	DESCRIPTION
DN	Referring Provider	The physician who requests the service for the patient.
DK	Ordering Provider	A physician or, when appropriate, a non-physician who orders non-physician services for the patient. These services include diagnostic laboratory tests, clinical laboratory tests, pharmaceutical services, or durable medical equipment.
DQ	Supervising Provider	The physician monitoring the patient's care.

BLOCK 17A Leave blank.

BLOCK 17B The NPI number goes here. As part of the enrollment process, all providers must apply for an NPI number. Authorized under the HIPAA Simplification Rule, the NPI is a unique identification number for all HIPAA-covered entities, including individuals, organizations, home health agencies, clinics, nursing homes, residential treatment homes, laboratories, ambulances, group practices, and health maintenance organizations (HMOs).

BLOCK 18 Dates entered in a six- or eight-digit format when a medical service rendered is a result of, or subsequent to, a related hospitalization.

FIGURE 4.7 *CMS-1500 Form Blocks 19-23*

Source: National Uniform Claim Committee

BLOCK 19 This block is used in numerous ways, based on the circumstances and payer type. Some common examples include:

- When modifier 99 (multiple modifiers) is used in block 24D, an explanation is given here in block 19 (e.g., 99 = 52 80 LT).

- When a claim needs to have a report or other documentation attached, enter "Additional Claim Information" in this block.

- Some payers require qualifiers in this block. Check with your private payer to see if this is required. NUCC provides a complete list on its website.

- Worker's Compensation requires additional information in this block. Each state has an official website for Worker's Compensation, with claim form instructions. NUCC also lists the qualifiers used.

- Medicare also has specific instructions for various situations and specialty claims. Complete instructions can be found at www.cms.gov.

BLOCK 20 Mark "yes" to the question asked if lab tests were done by an entity other than the one doing the billing. If multiple tests are involved, each should be filed under a separate claim.

BLOCK 21   This is where the diagnosis codes go.

BLOCK 22   Carrier-specific block; use for Medicaid claims.

BLOCK 23   The quality improvement organization (QIO) prior authorization number goes here for those procedures that require it. Enter the investigational device exemption (IDE) when an investigation device is used in an FDA-approved clinical trial.

Other information entered here includes the following.

- NPI of a home health agency or hospice when either is billed

- 10-digit Clinical Laboratory Improvement Act (CLIA) certification number for laboratory services billed by an entity performing CLIA-covered procedures

- ZIP code of a loaded ambulance's point of pick-up

IMPORTANT: Only one of these conditions can be listed per claim. If more than one apply, separate claims need to be submitted.

FIGURE 4.8 *CMS-1500 Form Blocks 24A-J*

Source: National Uniform Claim Committee

BLOCK 24A   Dates of service are listed here. Enter "From" and "To" dates in either a MMDDYY or MMDDCCYY format. When "From" and "To" dates are shown for a series of identical services, list them as a series of days in column G.

BLOCK 24B   This is where places of service codes go. These must be HIPAA-compliant. Codes are shown as two-digit numbers. For example, "01" should be used for a pharmacy; 02 is an unassigned number; 03 is for a school; and 04 is for a homeless shelter. For a complete list of codes, search www.cms.gov.

BLOCK 24C   Carrier-specific block; used by Medicaid. Enter an "x" when billing for emergency services, or the claim may be reduced or denied.

BLOCK 24D   Enter procedures, services, and supplies. For this field, use CPT or HCPCS codes. These will be described in Chapter 5. This is also the place where *modifiers* go. Modifiers are additional information about types of services, such as surgical care or outpatient services. Modifiers are part of valid CPT or HCPCS codes.

BLOCK 24E   This field is for the diagnosis reference code, as shown in Block 21. This field matches the date of service to the procedures performed under the primary diagnosis code. Enter only one reference number per line. Do *not* enter the diagnosis code here.

BLOCK 24F   Enter the provider's billed charges for each service.

BLOCK 24G   Enter the number of days or units. This field is mostly used for multiple visits, units of supplies, anesthesia minutes, or oxygen volume. If only one service is performed, the number "1" must be entered.

BLOCK 24H Carrier-specific block. For Medicaid claims, refer to the Family Planning section of the Medicaid Providers Manual for detailed instructions.

BLOCK 24I Enter the ID qualifier 1C in the shaded portion.

BLOCK 24J Enter the provider's NPI in the unshaded portion.

FIGURE 4.9 *CMS-1500 Form Blocks 25-33A*

25. FEDERAL TAX I.D. NUMBER SSN EIN	26. PATIENT'S ACCOUNT NO.	27. ACCEPT ASSIGNMENT? (For govt. claims, see back) YES NO	28. TOTAL CHARGE $	29. AMOUNT PAID $	30. Rsvd for NUCC Use
31. SIGNATURE OF PHYSICIAN OR SUPPLIER INCLUDING DEGREES OR CREDENTIALS (I certify that the statements on the reverse apply to this bill and are made a part thereof.) SIGNED DATE	32. SERVICE FACILITY LOCATION INFORMATION a. NPI b.		33. BILLING PROVIDER INFO & PH # ( ) a. NPI b.		

NUCC Instruction Manual available at: www.nucc.org   **PLEASE PRINT OR TYPE**   APPROVED OMB-0938-1197 FORM 1500 (02-12)

Source: National Uniform Claim Committee

BLOCK 25 Enter the provider's or supplier's federal ID number or Social Security number and check the appropriate box.

BLOCK 26 Enter the patient's account number as assigned by the provider or supplier.

BLOCK 27 Check the appropriate box to indicate whether the provider or supplier accepts assignment of benefits. Be aware of which providers can only be paid on an assignment basis.

BLOCK 28 Enter total charges for all services.

BLOCK 29 For secondary claims only. Enter the total amount the patient's primary insurance paid.

BLOCK 30 Leave blank.

BLOCK 31 Enter the signature of the provider or the signature of an authorized representative.

BLOCK 32 Enter the name, address, and ZIP code of the facility where services were rendered.

BLOCK 32A Enter the NPI of the facility.

BLOCK 33 The provider's or supplier's billing name, address, ZIP code, and telephone number.

BLOCK 33A The NPI of the billing provider.

Healthcare Common Procedure Coding System (HCPCS). A group of codes and descriptors used to represent health care procedures, supplies, products, and services.

UB-04 Form

Also called CMS-1450, this form is for institutional claims. The following information must be filled in on this form:

Information About the Provider

- Name and address of the billing provider
- Address where payment should go if it's different from the address given above
- The facility's unique account number assigned to the patient, up to 20 alphanumeric characters (will be printed on the RA and will help you identify the patient)
- Medical record number assigned to patient's medical record by the provider. It can have up to 30 alphanumeric characters.

- The correct code to specify the type of bill being submitted (for example, to specify hospital, clinic, rehab facility, or provider)
- Federal tax ID number
- Time period covered
- The number of administrative days spent processing the patient's information

Information About the Patient

- Patient's name
- Patient's address
- Birth date
- Date of episode of care
- Hour of episode of care

- Type of admission, such as emergent or urgent
- Source of admission, such as from a provider or a clinic
- Time of discharge from care
- Patient discharge status, such as discharged to home in to a short-term facility

Documenting an Accident

- Coding describing the incident
- State where an accident occurred
- Date when the accident occurred
- Reason for visit
- Prospective Payment System (PPS) code number assigned to the claim
- External cause of injury code

- Principal procedure code and date
- Other procedure codes
- Attending provider name and identifiers
- Operating provider name and identifiers
- Other provider names and identifiers
- Provider signature

What is the difference between CMS-1500 and UB-04?

ANSWER: CMS-1500 is used to submit paper claims for Medicare. UB-04 is used for institutional claims.

SUMMARY

This chapter described the laws in place to protect patients' privacy. It also explained the role of OSHA in ensuring workplace safety, and the regulations in place to prevent fraud. The chapter ends with a description of how to fill out two key forms: CMS-1500 and UB-04.

The next chapter focuses on how to explain to patients their rights, insurance responsibilities, and procedures they might need.

CHAPTER DRILL QUESTIONS

HIPAA Guidelines

1. How does HIPAA protect patients?

2. True or False: When storing files, the minimum necessary is to keep the files turned to the wall so that they cannot be seen by those walking by.

3. What is a Notice of Privacy Practices?

    a. Statement protecting the provider from lawsuits

    b. Statement of the patient's diagnosis

    c. Statement explaining emergency preparedness

    d. Statement signed by the patient that describes how private health information is protected

4. With whom are covered entities allowed to share information?

5. When is a patient's privacy not protected?

6. What is an incidental disclosure?

OSHA Guidelines

7. What is OSHA's mission?

Center for Medicare/Medicaid Services (CMS) Guidelines

8. What are the consequences of fraud?

9. What is the difference between Medicare and Medicaid?

10. What are three things that must be in an emergency preparedness plan?

CHAPTER DRILL ANSWERS

1. Answer: HIPAA protects patients by giving them more control over their medical records; authorizing them to make informed choices about the uses of their PHI; setting boundaries on the use and release of health records; establishing safeguards that providers must follow to ensure that the privacy of health information is protected; holding violators accountable if patients' privacy is compromised through both civil and criminal penalties; and protecting the balance struck between public health concerns and the disclosure of PHI.

2. Answer: True. This system helps protect other patients or medical staff not involved from seeing a patient's name, thus protecting that person's privacy.

3. **A.** INCORRECT: This kind of information would be included on a legal document, such as a deposition.
   B. INCORRECT: This type of information is included in specific codes.
   C. INCORRECT: This type of information is included in emergency procedures.
   D. CORRECT: The Privacy Rule provides that an individual has a right to adequate notice of how a covered entity may use and disclose protected health information about the individual. Some info is disclosed without permission. This is part of the notice.

4. Answer: According to the Privacy Rule, covered entities are allowed to share information relevant to the patient's care with a spouse, family member, friend, or other individual identified by the patient. The covered entity is also allowed to share relevant information if it can reasonably be inferred, based on professional judgment, that the patient does not object or that the action is in the patient's best interest.

5. Answer: A patient's privacy is not protected if access to records from a nursing home are needed to ensure that the providers are caring for the residents properly and the facility is clean; when there is a need to protect the public from epidemic or cases of sexually transmitted diseases (STDs) or cases of HIV/AIDS; when police reports about a gunshot wound are required; or when there are concerns about child abuse.

6. Answer: Incidental disclosure is secondary use that cannot be reasonably prevented, is limited in nature, and occurs as a result of another use or disclosure that is permitted. These kinds of disclosures are permitted under HIPAA.

7. Answer: OSHA's mission is to protect the health and safety of everyone in the workplace.

8. Answer: The OIG has the authority to exclude individuals and entities who have engaged in fraud and abuse from participating in Medicare, Medicaid, and other federal health care programs. The office also can impose penalties on offenders. The OIG keeps an office List of Excluded Individuals/Entities (LEIE).

9. Answer: Medicare is insurance for individuals 65 and older or for those under age 65 with disabilities. Medicaid is for those considered medically indigent; states must work with the federal government to ensure eligibility criteria.

10. Answer: An emergency preparedness plan should include information about how to inform patients and employees about an emergency, how to evacuate, and who should be left behind to monitor critical equipment before evacuating.

CHAPTER 5
Patient Education

OVERVIEW

Going to the doctor can be an overwhelming experience. Usually there are forms to fill out, and most people feel some anxiety about the visit. On top of that, people can feel that they don't have much control over the situation.

In reality, patients have many rights when it comes to their medical care. These have been compiled in a list referred to as the *Patient's Bill of Rights*. This chapter explains the different elements of this important document.

With rights come responsibilities. For patients, this includes meeting insurance responsibilities. This chapter also goes over what insurance terms patients need to understand to meet their obligations. The chapter ends with information patients need when preparing for a medical procedure.

By the end of this chapter, you should be able to answer the following questions.

1. Why was the Patient's Bill of Rights established?
2. True or False: Patients have no choice in the providers they see.
3. What is not included in the Patient's Bill of Rights?
4. What is abandonment?
5. What is informed consent?
6. True or False: Consent is required for minors in a life-threatening situation.
7. What is a deductible?
8. What is an explanation of benefits (EOB)?
9. What is the difference between Medicare and Medicaid?
10. What information does the patient need before undergoing a medical test or procedure?

PATIENT'S BILL OF RIGHTS

Introduction

In 1998, President Clinton created the President's Advisory Commission on Consumer Protection and Quality in the Healthcare Industry. The purpose of the commission was to make recommendations to ensure that patients receive high-quality health care. From this work emerged a document called the Consumer Bill of Rights and Responsibilities, referred to as the Patient's Bill of Rights.

The document is designed to accomplish the following goals.

- To strengthen consumer confidence by ensuring that the health care system is fair and responsive to consumer's needs, provides them with credible, effective mechanisms for addressing their concerns, and encourages them to take an active role in improving and ensuring their health

- To reaffirm the importance of a strong relationship between patients and their health care professionals

- To reaffirm the critical role consumers play in safeguarding their health by establishing rights and responsibilities for all participants in improving their health

This information may be presented to patients when they are admitted to a health care facility or come to the office for treatment. Some offices post them in a prominent place. It is the job of the medical administrative assistant to explain procedures to patients and to make sure they provide written consent. The next section explains this process in more detail.

Patient's Bill of Rights. A list of guarantees for people receiving medical care

The Eights Points of the Patient's Bill of Rights

The first step for the medical administrative assistant is becoming familiar with the Patient's Bill of Rights. It includes the following eight points.

1. Information Disclosure

Patients have a right to receive accurate, easily understood information about their health plan, health care professionals, and health care facilities. If the patient speaks another language, has a physical or mental disability, or doesn't understand something, assistance will be provided so that the patient can make informed health care decisions.

2. Choice of Providers and Plans

Patients have the right to a choice of providers sufficient to provide access to appropriate, high-quality health care.

3. Access to Emergency Services

If a patient has severe pain, an injury, or a sudden illness that convinces that individual that his or her health is in serious jeopardy, the patient has the right to receive screening and stabilization emergency services whenever and wherever needed, without prior authorization or financial penalty.

4. Participation in Treatment Decisions

Patients have the right to know all their treatment options and to participate in decisions about their care. Parents, guardians, family members, or other individuals designated by patients can represent them if they cannot make their own decisions.

5. Respect and Nondiscrimination

Patients have the right to considerate, respectful, and nondiscriminatory care from providers and health plan representatives.

6. Confidentiality of Health Information

While providers own the medical records, patients have the right to talk in confidence with providers and to have their health care information protected. Patients also have the right to review and copy their own medical record and request that the provider amend the record if it is not accurate, relevant, or complete.

7. Complaints and Appeals

Patients have the right to a fair, fast, and objective review of any complaint against the health plan, providers, hospitals, or other health care personnel. This includes complaints about waiting times, operating hours, the conduct of health care personnel, and the adequacy of health care facilities.

8. Consumer Responsibilities

In a health care system that protects consumer rights, it is reasonable to expect and encourage consumers to assume reasonable responsibilities. Greater individual involvement by consumers in their care increases the likelihood of achieving the best outcomes and help support a quality-improvement, cost-conscious environment.

Explaining the Patient's Bill of Rights

Each of these points must be explained to the patient. The following section presents a more detailed discussion of topics that must be covered.

Information Disclosure. For English-speaking patients, this means having brochures, fact sheets, and other materials available to give to patients to help them understand their medical condition and treatment options. For non-English speakers and those who have disabilities, the Americans with Disabilities Act (ADA) says that accommodations must be made so that communication can take place. This involves having educational materials available in the predominant language(s) spoken in the community; having materials in Braille; and having access to a sign language interpreter.

Choice of Providers and Plans. Make sure that patients are aware that depending on their health plans, there can be some limitations on their choice of providers. For example, some health plans require that patients choose providers from a network, and some networks are more extensive than others. But if the patient likes the provider, she has the right to continue seeing that person. Similarly, if the patient would like to switch providers, that is allowed, too. If the patient wants or needs to see a specialist, she has that right and might need a *referral* from your office. A referral tells the specialist that the patient is authorized to be treated.

Access to Emergency Services. Check your office's policies about emergency treatment. There may be some referral requirements, or the patient's health plan may have restrictions. Make sure the patient is aware of the procedures in place for emergency services.

Participation in Treatment Decisions. In the past, providers were viewed as the source of all medical knowledge and made the decisions for patients. But that is changing. In recent years, there has been a trend toward *shared decision-making.* This means that the patient and provider work together to decide on a treatment plan. Shared decision-making is another reason patients need access to information.

A related scenario involved the provider's obligations to patients once a relationship has been established. If a provider decides to stop seeing a patient, he must give the patient sufficient time to find another provider. Also, the provider should write a letter of withdrawal from medical care and have it delivered by certified mail, with a return receipt requested. The letter must state that professional care is being discontinued; that the provider will give copies of the patient's records to another provider on request; and that the patient should seek the care of another provider as soon as possible.

A copy of this letter and the return receipt should be put in the patient's medical record and permanently retained. The patient should be given a reasonable amount of time to find another provider.

referral. Written recommendation to a specialist.

shared decision-making. A patient and provider work together to decide on a treatment plan.

The provider must be careful to follow these rules. Otherwise, he could be vulnerable to a lawsuit for *abandonment*, or discontinuing medical care without giving the proper notice. If a patient wants to terminate care with the provider, she doesn't have to inform the office. But if the patient chooses to inform the office manager, then a letter confirming the termination of the relationship is usually requested.

> *abandonment.* Discontinuing medical care without giving the proper notice or providing a competent replacement.

- *Respect and Nondiscrimination.* Review the office policy on discrimination to make sure that it is designed to treat every patient with respect. All employees must be courteous and considerate to every patient and visitor.

- *Confidentiality of Health Information.* Explain to patients that their health information is confidential, and the medical practice will do everything possible to ensure that their confidentiality is respected. Also, explain that their records belong to the medical practice, but they also the right to see their records. Often this involves submitting a request in writing.

- *Complaints and Appeals.* Give patients information about how to submit complaints and file grievances.

- *Consumer Responsibilities.* Both providers and patients bear some responsibilities in ensuring that the best quality of care is given. For providers, this means working with other staff members to make sure that the office maintains the highest level of quality while remaining cost-conscious. For patients, it means becoming knowledgeable about their health so that they can be active partners in their care. This should result in the best, most cost-effective treatment.

In all interactions with patients, the medical staff must be sensitive to patients' needs and desires. To achieve this goal, the staff must understand the Patient's Bill of Rights and incorporate it into all their dealings with patients.

Since ACA was passed, the following points were added to the Patient's Bill of Rights.

- *Ban on Discriminating Against Children with Pre-existing Conditions.* Before reform, insurance companies could deny a family insurance because of a child's pre-existing illness or disorder. After 2014, this practice is allowed.

- *Ban on Insurance Companies Dropping Coverage.* Previously, insurance companies could drop consumers, even if they were very sick, due to a mistake on their application. This is no longer permitted.

- *Ban on Insurance Companies Limiting Coverage.* Previously, there was a cap on the amount of coverage insurance companies would pay over a person's lifetime. For those suffering from a chronic disease, this could mean that insurance could be cut off. This is no longer allowed. Beginning in 2014, annual limits for all forms of health care—hospital, provider, and pharmacy—also are banned. Insurance companies will no longer be able to restrict the dollars spent on healthcare each year.

- *Ban on Insurance Companies Limiting Choice of Providers.* Insurance companies are no longer able to determine which providers patients choose. Patients can now choose their own providers within the plan's network.

- *Ban on Restricting Emergency Room Care.* Insurance carriers can no longer determine where patients go for emergency care or charge more if they go out of network.

- *Guarantee Patient's Right to Appeal.* Previously, consumers had few options if an insurance carrier denied or restricted treatment. Now they are guaranteed the right to appeal.

- *Coverage for Young Adults.* Beginning in 2010, adult children can stay on their parents' health insurance plan up to the age of 26. This applies to married and unmarried children and is an option even if the young adults are offered health insurance through an employer.

- *Covering Preventive Care at No Cost.* Preventive care, such as mammograms, colonoscopies, immunizations, and prenatal and new baby care, are provided at no cost to consumers.

What are two points in the Patient's Bill of Rights?

ANSWER: The right to receive accurate, easy-to-understand information about their insurance plan, provider, and health care facilities. As much as possible given any constraints in the health plan, the right to choose providers.

What are two points that have been added to the Patient's Bill of Rights since the ACA was passed?

ANSWER: The right to appeal insurance carriers' restriction on care and coverage of young adults up to age 26.

Kinds of Consent

Before treating patients, providers must have their permission, or *consent.* For routine care, consent is usually implied when the patient comes to the office for care. This kind of consent, called *implied consent,* is sufficient for common or simple procedures that typically involve little risk. Blood-drawing, or phlebotomy, and taking vital signs, such as blood pressure and temperature, fall under this category.

In some instances, it is sufficient to receive *verbal* consent. This kind of consent is considered more direct than implicit consent, because it is said out loud in response to a pointed question. It does not, however, have the legal clout of *informed consent,* which providers must get for more complex procedures. Informed consent involves making sure the patient has a full understanding of her condition and enough information to make a sound decision about treatment options. Therefore, a conversation must be held between the patient or the patient's legal representative, presenting the necessary information.

According to the American Medical Association (AMA), the conversation should include the following elements.

- Patient's diagnosis, if known

- Nature and purpose of the propose treatment or procedure

- Risks and benefits of the proposed treatment or procedure

- Alternative treatments or procedures, regardless of the cost or the extent to which the treatment options are covered by health insurance

- Risks and benefits of the alternative treatment (or treatments) and procedure (or procedures)

- Risks and benefits of not receiving or undergoing a treatment or procedure

implied consent. A patient presents for treatment, such as extending an arm to allow a venipuncture to be performed.

verbal consent. Consent for treatment given out loud in response to a pointed question.

informed consent. Providers explain medical or diagnostic procedures, surgical interventions, and the benefits and risks involved, giving patients an opportunity to ask questions and consent before medical intervention is provided.

This conversation must be held with the provider, not the medical administrative assistant, and it must be fully documented. The medical administrative assistant's role is to present the informed consent document to the patient and witness it as the patient signs it. Furthermore, each state has its own consent laws, which the medical administrative assistant should become familiar with.

There are legal consequences to not following the laws surrounding informed consent. If a provider doesn't get informed consent, he could be charged with the crime of *assault and battery*, which is willful and unlawful use of force or violence on another person.

If an individual is found to be incompetent for reason of insanity or another issue, that individual usually cannot give consent for medical treatment. Consent then must be obtained from a guardian.

---

assault and battery. Willful and unlawful use of intimidation and physical force or violence on another person.

Why is informed consent important?

ANSWER: Informed consent is based on the patient's understanding of the reason for a particular treatment plan. It is the job of the provider and medical staff to ensure that the patient reaches this level of understanding. Then the patient is asked to sign a consent form, which confirms this understanding and allows the patient to make a thoughtful decision based on the facts. Informed consent also protects the provider against the crime of assault and battery.

Consent for Minors

When the patient is a minor, consent for surgery or treatment must be obtained from a parent or guardian, except in an emergency situation. If the parents are legally separated or divorced, then consent must come from the custodial parent. If the child is visiting the other parent, consent can be obtained from that parent, because that parent has temporary custody.

Consent is not required for minors under the following circumstances.

- When consent may be implied, such as in a life-threatening situation.

- When a certain treatment is required by law, such as a vaccination or an x-ray for school entry or safety.

- When a court order has been issued if parents have withheld consent for what is considered a necessary treatment for religious reasons.

- In many states, treatment for sexually transmitted diseases, drug abuse, alcohol dependency, pregnancy, or providing birth control does not require consent from parents.

In some instances, minors are considered emancipated. In these instances, parental consent is not required. An *emancipated minor* is a person younger than the age of majority (usually 18, but up to 21 in some states) who is:

- Married.

- In the armed forces.

- Living apart from parents or a guardian.

- Self-supporting.

---

emancipated minor. A person younger than the age of majority (usually 18 to 21 years of age) who is married, in the armed forces, living apart from parents or a guardian, or self-supporting.

PATIENT INSURANCE RESPONSIBILITIES

Health insurance is designed to help individuals and patients offset the costs of medical care. It is defined as protection against financial losses resulting from illness or injury. Health insurance covers services and procedures considered medically necessary.

The patient bears financial responsibilities in the form of copayments, coinsurance, and deductibles. *Copayments* are a fixed dollar amount that must be paid each time a patient visits a provider. Copayments may vary from provider to provider. A visit to an outpatient clinic might have a $15 copay, while the copay for outpatient surgery might be $50.

Coinsurance is the pre-established percentage of expenses paid by the insurance company after the deductible has been met. Many plans have an 80-20 formula in place, meaning that the insurance company pays 80% of the costs and the member pays 20%. For example, if a cost of a medical service is $500, the insurance company $400 and the member pays $100.

Deductibles refer to the amount of money patients must pay out of pocket before the insurance company will start to pay for covered benefits. Deductibles vary considerably from plan to plan. The deductible must be met for each calendar year. Any expenses not covered will be applied to the deductible.

There are also limits for how much of the cost of a procedure will be reimbursed by the insurance company. This is called the *allowable amount,* or the maximum amount of money many third-party payers (both government and private insurance companies) allow for a given procedure or service. This amount is either written off by the provider or passed on to the patient. The *explanation of benefits (EOB),* which the patient receives from the insurance carrier, will identify what was paid, reduced, or denied, as well as the deductible, coinsurance, and allowable amount. Medicare patients receive a similar document called the *Medicare Summary Notice (MSN).* Both documents prepare the patient for what bills to expect.

FIGURE 5.1 *Explanation of benefits*

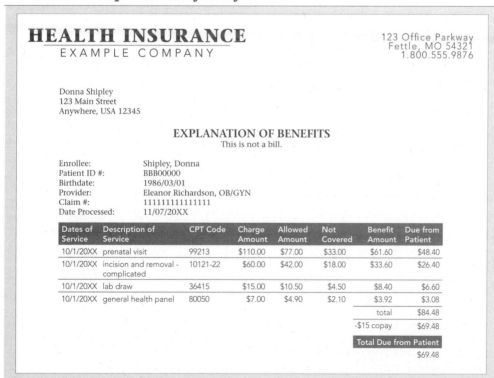

HEALTH INSURANCE
EXAMPLE COMPANY

123 Office Parkway
Fettle, MO 54321
1.800.555.9876

Donna Shipley
123 Main Street
Anywhere, USA 12345

EXPLANATION OF BENEFITS
This is not a bill.

Enrollee: Shipley, Donna
Patient ID #:   BBB00000
Birthdate: 1986/03/01
Provider: Eleanor Richardson, OB/GYN
Claim #:   111111111111111
Date Processed: 11/07/20XX

Dates of Service	Description of Service	CPT Code	Charge Amount	Allowed Amount	Not Covered	Benefit Amount	Due from Patient
10/1/20XX	prenatal visit	99213	$110.00	$77.00	$33.00	$61.60	$48.40
10/1/20XX	incision and removal - complicated	10121-22	$60.00	$42.00	$18.00	$33.60	$26.40
10/1/20XX	lab draw	36415	$15.00	$10.50	$4.50	$8.40	$6.60
10/1/20XX	general health panel	80050	$7.00	$4.90	$2.10	$3.92	$3.08
						total	$84.48
						-$15 copay	$69.48
						Total Due from Patient	
							$69.48

Medicare Summary Notice (MSN). Document that outlines all of the services and supplies, the amounts billed by the provider, the amounts paid by Medicare, and what the patient must pay the provider for the preceding 3-month period.

private health insurance. Health insurance subsidized through premiums paid directly to the company.

Finally, many plans have a maximum in place. That means that after the members have reached a predetermined amount, the insurance company will pay 100% of the cost of the medical service. For example, a health plan could establish $5,000 as its maximum amount. A patient covered by that plan who has a major surgery would pay out of pocket up to $5,000, but nothing after that.

What's the difference between a copayment and coinsurance?

ANSWER: A copayment is a flat fee that a patient pays for visiting a provider or purchasing prescription drugs. The copayment can vary from provider to provider. Coinsurance is a percentage of the covered benefits paid by both the insurance company and the patient. Many insurance companies pay 80% of the covered benefits, with the patient paying the remaining 20%.

GOVERNMENT AND PRIVATE INSURANCE

Introduction

People have several options for health insurance. The government offers health plans for specialized audiences. Medicare is mostly for people age 65 and older, with some exceptions. Medicaid is for families and individuals with disabilities or limited financial resources.

However, most people get their insurance through commercial sources. They can purchase *private insurance* through an insurance company. Their health care is subsidized through premiums paid directly to the company.

Another option is to get health insurance through employers. If these plans are *self-insured* by the employer, they tend to be lower-cost because additional fees are not built into the premiums. The employers budget a certain amount for employees' claims, which employers pay as they come in. However, some employers purchase group plans for their employees.

The ACA has given individuals and families another place to go for health insurance: the Federal Insurance Marketplace. Opened in October 2013, the Marketplace is designed to provide consumers with an online place to go to shop for health insurance. Consumers can compare plans in their area, get answers to questions, and find out if they are eligible for tax credits, which are available for private and some government insurance plans. Some states have marketplaces set up where consumers can shop as well.

The Small Business Health Options Program (SHOP) opened in 2014. Like the marketplace for consumers, SHOP provides small businesses with a streamlined opportunity to purchase high-quality health insurance for their employees. There is no open enrollment for this service, so small-business employers can buy health insurance throughout the year.

premium. A pre-established amount set by the insurance company and paid regularly, usually on a monthly basis, by the patient or an employer.

Government Insurance

Medicare

Medicare is health insurance provided to people 65 years of age or older, people younger than 65 with certain disabilities, and all people who have end-stage kidney disease.

Medicare has the following four parts.

Medicare Part A provides hospitalization insurance generally free of charge to individuals eligible for the Medicare benefit. Health care services covered include inpatient hospital care, skilled nursing facility care, home health care, hospice care, and inpatient care in a religious, non-medical health care institution. Inpatient hospital coverage and coverage for skilled nursing facility care are measured in *benefit periods*. A benefit period begins when the patient is admitted to a hospital or skilled nursing facility and ends when the patient has not received care for 60 days in a row. There are certain limitations on how much coverage Medicare Part A pays for each kind of service.

Under *Medicare Part B,* people can purchase voluntary supplemental medical insurance (SMI) to help pay for providers' and other medical professionals' services, medical services, and medical-surgical supplies not covered by Medicare Part A. Other services covered include care provided at an emergency department, or an outpatient clinic, such as same-day surgery; home health care not covered under Part A; laboratory tests, x-rays, and other diagnostic radiology services; ambulatory surgery center services at Medicare-approved facilities; most physical, speech, and occupational therapy services; radiation therapy, kidney dialysis, and transplants; heart and liver transplants; and inpatient hospitalizations when Part A benefits have been exhausted.

Services not covered by Part A or Part B include the following.

- Long-term nursing care
- Cosmetic surgery
- Dentures and dental care
- Acupuncture
- Hearing aids and exams for fitting hearing aids

Medicare. Federally funded health insurance provided to people age 65 or older, people younger than 65 who have certain disabilities, and people of all ages with end-stage kidney disease.

---

benefit period. Time during which benefits are payable under a given insurance plan.

Medicare Part A. Provides hospitalization insurance to eligible individuals.

Medicare Part B. Voluntary supplemental medical insurance to help pay for physicians' and other medical professionals' services, medical services, and medical-surgical supplies not covered by Medicare Part A.

Medicare Advantage (MA) plans offer a combined package of the benefits under both Parts A and B. In some instances, they offer extra coverage for services such as vision, hearing, dental, or health and wellness programs. Many also include prescription drug coverage. Organizations offering MA plans must meet specific requirements from CMS.

Medicare Advantage (MA). Combined package of benefits under Medicare Parts A and B that may offer extra coverage for services such as vision, hearing, dental, health and wellness, or prescription drug coverage.

---

health maintenance organization (HMO). Plan that allows patients to only go to physicians, other health care professionals, or hospitals on a list of approved providers, except in an emergency.

---

preferred provider organization (PPO). Plan that allows patients to use physicians, specialists, and hospitals in the plan's network and receive a greater discount on services.

---

private fee-for-service plan. Plan that allows patients to go to any physician, other health care professional, or hospital as long as the providers agree to treat those patients.

---

fee-for-service. Model in which providers set the fees for procedures and services.

Advance Beneficiary Notice of Noncoverage (ABN). Form provided to a patient if a provider believes that a service may be declined because Medicare might consider it unnecessary.

Medicare Part D. A plan run by private insurance companies and other vendors approved by Medicare to cover the cost of approved prescriptions.

---

out-of-pocket maximum. A predetermined amount after which the insurance company will pay 100% of the cost of medical services.

The following options are available through Medicare Advantage.

- *Health maintenance organizations (HMOs)* allow patients to only go to providers, other health care professionals, or hospitals on the plan's list of approved providers, except in an emergency.

- *Preferred provider organizations (PPOs)* allow patients to use doctors, specialists, and hospitals in the plan's network. Going to doctors and hospitals not on the list usually means that patients will have to pay extra.

- *Private fee-for-service plans* allow patients to go to any doctor, other health care professional, or hospital as long as the providers agree to treat those patients. The plan determines how much it will pay providers and how much patients must pay for care. People enrolled in Medicare may receive an *Advance Beneficiary Notice of Noncoverage (ABN)* if there is a possibility that Medicare will deny coverage. Items that may fall into this category include certain Part A (hospice care or home health agencies) and Part B (outpatient) services. Your office may send out an ABN if there is concern that Medicare won't cover a particular service; if Medicare usually pays for that service; or if Medicare may not consider the particular service medically necessary for a particular patient in a particular plan. This form also may be used to alert patients to services that Medicare never covers.

- *Medicare specialty plans* provide focused, specialized health care for specific groups of people, such as those who have both Medicare and Medicaid, live in a nursing home, or have chronic medical conditions.

Medicare Part D pays for medications. The drug benefit is run by private insurance companies and other vendors approved by Medicare. There are many plans to choose from, and they can vary in cost and drugs covered. Beneficiaries can choose the plan that best meets their needs.

Out-of-pocket expenses mostly come up for people who choose the fee-for-service option. They are responsible for charges not covered by Medicare, as well as for various cost-sharing requirements of Parts A and B. These expenses may be paid by the Medicare beneficiary, an employer-sponsored health, or *Medigap,* a private health insurance that pays for most of the charges not covered by Parts A and B. If a beneficiary is eligible for Medicaid, it could pay for some of the outstanding expenses not covered by Medicare.

Medicaid

This government-based health insurance option is funded through a partnership between state governments and the federal Medicaid program. The program pays for medical assistance for individuals who have low incomes and limited financial resources.

To participate in Medicaid, states must meet national guidelines established by federal laws, regulations, and policies. If the states meet those requirements, they qualify for federal matching grants. Each state has its own agency that determines Medicaid eligibility for its residents. Medicaid policies vary from state to state, so a person eligible in one state might not be eligible in another. However, the federal government has established that the following are considered *categorically needy eligible groups*.

Medicaid. A government-based health insurance option that pays for medical assistance for individuals who have low incomes and limited financial resources. Funded at the state and national level. Administered at the state level.

- Those who meet the requirements for Temporary Assistance for Needy Families (TANF)
- Children below the age of 6 whose family income is at or below 133% of the federal poverty level
- Pregnant women whose family income is below 133% of the federal poverty level
- Supplemental Security Income recipients (in most states)
- Recipients of adoption or foster care assistance
- Individuals who lose their cash assistance due to earnings from work or increased Social Security benefits
- Infants born to Medicaid-eligible women
- Certain low-income Medicare recipients

Services Covered Under Medicaid

To receive federal matching funds, Medicaid must provide medical assistance for the following services.

- Inpatient hospital care
- Outpatient hospital care
- Emergency care
- Prenatal care
- Vaccines for children
- Providers' services
- Skilled nursing facilities services for persons aged 2 or older
- Family planning services and supplies
- Rural health clinic services
- Home health care for persons eligible for skilled nursing services
- Laboratory and x-ray services
- Pediatric and family nurse practitioner services
- Nurse-midwife services
- Federally qualified health center services and ambulatory services performed at a federally qualified health center that would be available in other settings
- Early and periodic screening, diagnosis, and therapeutic services for children under age 21

States may also receive federal matching funds to provide some of the following optional services.

- Diagnostic services
- Clinic services
- Prescription drugs and prosthetic devices
- Transportation services
- Rehabilitation and physical therapy services
- Home care and community-based care services for people who have chronic impairments

State Children's Health Insurance Program (SCHIP)

This program is also jointly funded by the federal government and the states. States must meet the following three eligibility criteria.

- Recipients must come from low-income families.

- Recipients must be otherwise ineligible for Medicaid.

- Recipients must be uninsured.

States must offer the following services.

- Inpatient hospital care

- Outpatient hospital care

- Providers' surgical and medical services

- Laboratory and x-ray services

- Well baby/child care, including age-appropriate immunizations

---

State Children's Health Insurance Program (SCHIP). A program jointly funded by the federal government and the states to cover uninsured children in families with modest incomes too high to qualify for Medicaid.

Commercial Insurance

This term refers to three kinds of insurance: Individual, employer-sponsored, and employer-based self-insurance. *Individual insurance plans* are paid for by the individual, while *employer-based self-insurance* is tied to an individual's place of employment. Both kinds of commercial insurance are explained in the following sections.

Individual Health Insurance Plans

These plans are paid for through premiums, which are a pre-established amount set by the insurance company and paid regularly, usually on a monthly basis. The premiums of all the plan's participants go into a fund, which is used to pay for claims. Before paying a claim, the company reviews it carefully to make sure the service is covered by the plan. They also check the diagnosis codes to make sure the services were medically necessary. Payment is made to either the provider or the policyholder.

Upfront information provided to the policyholder before signing on to a plan includes the following.

- What medical services will be covered

- When the company will pay for those medical services

- How much and for how long the company will pay for the covered services

- Which process must be followed to ensure that covered medical expenses are paid

Moving forward, some patients may say that they have plans through "Obamacare." What they really mean is that they purchased a plan through a carrier, such as Aetna or Blue Cross and Blue Shield, on the ACA marketplace. Those plans will likely fit a *managed care model*. Managed care refers to plans that provide care in return for preset, scheduled payments and that coordinate health care through a network of primary care providers (PCPs), hospitals, and other providers. The next section describes two common types of managed care plans: health maintenance organizations (HMOs) and preferred provider organizations (PPOs).

managed care organization. Organization developed to manage the quality of health care and control costs.

Health Maintenance Organizations

HMOs provide comprehensive healthcare to an enrolled group for a fixed period of time. Some of these plans pay by *capitation,* meaning that the provider is paid a fixed amount for each individual enrolled in the plan during a specific period of time, regardless of the expense or number of services provided to the patient.

There are pros and cons to managed care. The pros are that health care costs usually are contained; established fee schedules are used; authorized services are compensated; and patients' out-of-pocket expenses tend to be less that they would be with traditional insurance.

capitation. The fixed amount a provider receives.

The cons are that access to specialized care can be limited; physicians' choices in the treatment of patients can be limited; the paperwork can be greater; and treatment might be delayed due to preauthorization requirements.

preauthorization. Formal approval from the insurance company that it will cover the test or procedure.

For these reasons, it is important for the medical administrative assistant to understand which services are covered, which are not, and which require special forms for billing. With this information in hand, the medical administrative assistant can explain covered benefits to patients and that steps that must be taken for procedures and services requiring preapproval.

Preferred Provider Organizations

Under this model, an insurer representing clients (an individual or a business) contracts with a group of providers who agree on a predetermined list of charges for all services. These include both normal and complex procedures. Unlike HMOs, PPOs have no capitation or prepaid care. These plans usually have deductibles and/or coinsurance payments of 20% to 25%. The insurer then pays the balance.

preferred provider organization (PPO). Plan that allows patients to use physicians, specialists, and hospitals in the plan's network and receive a greater discount on services.

Providers like this model because it preserves the fee-for-service approach, where the provider is reimbursed for the care given. When a patient is covered under a PPO plan, the provider treats the patient and bills the PPO.

To choose providers, subscribers are given a list of those in the network. Rates of those providers are typically lower than those outside the network. Therefore, if a patient goes to an out-of-network provider, the out-of-pocket costs will be higher.

Employer-Based Self-Insurance Plans

The idea behind employed-based self-insurance plans is that companies save money by self-insuring their employee health plans rather than purchasing coverage from private insurance companies. Self-insurance costs are lower because additional fees built into premiums by private insurers are eliminated.

employer-based insurance. Insurance that is tied to an individual's place of employment.

administrative services only (ASO) contract. Contract between employers and private insurers under which employers fund the plans themselves, and the private insurers administer the plans for the employers.

Employer-based self-insurance plans vary in their design and what services are covered. Many have a cost-sharing feature, where expenses are shared with employees and are taken out of their paychecks each pay period. But because of economies of scale, costs of employer-based health insurance plans tend to be lower than those purchased by individuals.

Plans usually are funded through *administrative services only (ASO) contracts* between employers and private insurers. Under these contracts, employers fund the plans themselves, and the private insurers administer the plans for the employers.

Blue Cross and Blue Shield Plans

These plans were the first prepaid plans in the United States. Originally, Blue Cross covered hospital care and Blue Shield covered providers' services. They merged to form the Blue Cross and Blue Shield Association (BC/BS) in 1982.

Blue Cross and Blue Shield plan. The first prepaid plan in the U.S. that offers health insurance to individuals, small businesses, seniors, and large employer groups.

BC/BS, also called the Blues, includes more than 60 independent, locally operated companies with plans in 50 states, the District of Columbia, and Puerto Rico. BC/BS offers health insurance to individuals, small businesses, seniors, and large employer groups. The federal government also has a large program called the BC/BS Federal Employee Program.

How does the government help with health insurance?

ANSWER: The government provides Medicare, Medicaid, and State Children's Health Insurance Program (SCHIP), and offers health insurance options on the marketplace through the Affordable Care Act.

What is the difference between individual health insurance and employer self-insured plans?

ANSWER: Private health insurance is paid by individuals or employers in the form of premiums to the insurance company. Employer self-insured plans are purchased in bulk by the employer and are generally more cost-effective. Additional costs embedded in premiums are largely eliminated, and employers fund the health insurance plans. Often employers enter into agreements with private insurers to manage the plans.

PRE- AND POST-INSTRUCTIONS FOR TESTING AND PROCEDURES

Medical administrative assistants often are asked to arrange outpatient diagnostic testing and procedures. Testing can include magnetic resonance imaging (MRI), computed tomography (CT) scans, x-ray evaluations, ultrasound testing, and blood tests. Possible procedures include dilation and curettage (D&C) and biopsies.

When setting up appointments for diagnostic testing or procedures, take the following steps.

1. Obtain a written order from the provider that describes the exact procedure to be performed. If a referral is needed, make sure you have a copy of that. This paperwork provides the necessary documentation for the test or procedure.

2. If the patient's insurance requires preauthorization, make sure to take care of this. Preauthorization involves notifying the health insurance plan that a patient needs a procedure, giving the insurance company the opportunity to determine whether the procedure is medically necessary. This will ensure that the insurance benefits are valid and will cover the patient's medical needs.

3. Make sure the patient is available at the time the test or procedure has been scheduled. If the provider needs to be there, make sure she is available as well.

4. Confirm that the diagnostic facility is a participating provider with the patient's insurance company. Then call the facility and schedule the patient's procedure or test. Remember to follow these steps.

   a. Order the test.

   b. Provide the patient's diagnosis and orders.

   c. Establish the date and time for the procedure.

   d. Give the patient's name, age, address, and telephone number.

   e. Provide the patient's demographic information, including identification and insurance policy numbers, as well as addresses for filing claims.

   f. Determine any special instructions for the patient or special anesthesia requirements.

   g. Notify the facility of any urgency for test results.

5. Let the patient know about the arrangements. Make sure to inform the patient of the following.

   a. Name, address, and telephone number of the facility

   b. Date and time to report for the test

   c. Instructions for preparing for the test, including eating restrictions, fluid requirements, and whether medications should be taken

   d. Information about preadmission testing

   e. The need to bring a form of picture identification and insurance card to the facility on the day of the procedure

   f. Whether the patient needs to pick up orders or whether they will be forwarded to the facility in advance

   g. After going through the list, ask the patient to repeat the instructions. Also, remind the patient of the importance of keeping the appointment and arriving on time.

6. Have the provider review the consent form with the patient. The patient should sign the consent form, and a copy should be placed in his medical record. This process will ensure that the patient understands the risks, benefits, and alternatives to the procedure.

7. Document the information in the patient's chart. Then check the patient's status following the procedure. Make sure the patient is following the provider's post-procedure instructions. Follow up with the facility if results are not received promptly.

SUMMARY

The patient has a key role to play in his or her health care. This chapter identified what the patients' rights are, and emphasized the importance of explaining these rights to them. All patients, including those who have disabilities or language barriers, must be told of their rights in a way they can understand.

With rights, however, come responsibilities. The chapter also explains patients' financial responsibilities, which usually are in the form of copayments, coinsurance, and deductibles. The chapter ends with a discussion on the steps that must be followed to schedule procedures and tests and inform the patient of what he or she needs to do before and after the procedure.

The next chapter will revisit many of the ideas we have already discussed, but from the perspective of office practices that need to be performed on a regular basis.

CHAPTER DRILL QUESTIONS

Patient's Bill of Rights

1. Why was the Patient's Bill of Rights established?

2. True or False: Patients have no choice in the providers they see.

3. What is not included in the Patient's Bill of Rights?

    a. The right to expect reasonable information from the provider

    b. The right to expect information to be kept confidential

    c. The right to take home one's own medical record

    d. The right to a fair hearing about any complaint against a provider, health plan, or facility

Patient Insurance Responsibilities

4. What is abandonment?

5. What is informed consent?

6. True or False: Consent is required for minors in a life-threatening situation.

Government and Private Insurance

7. What is a deductible?

8. What is an explanation of benefits (EOB)?

    a. Explains what services Medicare will not cover

    b. The amount the patient pays after each visit

    c. A document that identifies what was paid, reduced, or denied

    d. The percentage of the premium that the patient must cover

9. What is the difference between Medicare and Medicaid?

Pre- and Post-Instructions for Testing and Procedures

10. What information does the patient need before undergoing a medical test or procedure?

CHAPTER DRILL ANSWERS

1. Answer: The Patient's Bill of Rights was established to strengthen consumer confidence by ensuring that the health care system is fair and responsive to consumers' needs, provides them with credible, effective mechanisms for addressing their concerns, and encourages them to take an active role in improving and ensuring their health; to reaffirm the importance of a strong relationship between patients and their health care professionals; and to reaffirm the critical role consumers play in safeguarding their health by establishing rights and responsibilities for all participants in improving their health.

2. Answer: False. Patients have the right to choose a provider, but they must follow any limitations set by their health insurance plan.

3. **A.** INCORRECT: This right is called information disclosure.
    B. INCORRECT: This is described in detail in the Patient's Bill of Rights.
    C. CORRECT: This is not a right in the Patient's Bill of Rights. The medical record belongs to the practice.
    D. INCORRECT: This is a right in the Patient's Bill of Rights.

4. Answer: Abandonment is when a provider discontinues medical care without giving the proper notice.

5. Answer: Informed consent is when a patient gives written approval for a procedure or test based on information presented by the provider. This process ensures that the patient is prepared to make a sound decision about her care.

6. Answer: False. This is one of four exceptions when consent for minors is not required.

7. Answer: A deductible refers to the amount of money patients must pay out of pocket before the insurance company will start to pay for covered benefits.

8. **A.** INCORRECT: This document is called an Advance Beneficiary Notice of Noncoverage (ABN).
    B. INCORRECT: This amount is the copayment.
    C. CORRECT: The patient receives an EOB from the insurance carrier. It identifies what was paid, reduced, or denied, as well as the deductible, coinsurance, and allowable amount..
    D. INCORRECT: This is a description of the patient's coinsurance responsibility.

9. Answer: Medicare is government-issued health insurance for people age 65 and older. Medicaid is another form of government insurance, but it is for people who have low incomes, limited financial resources, or disabilities.

10. Answer: The patient needs to know the date and time of the test; what to do to prepare for test, such as eating restrictions, fluid requirements, and whether medications should be taken; and information about preadmission testing. The patient also needs to bring a form of picture identification and insurance card to the facility on the day of the procedure. She needs to know whether she needs to pick up orders or if they will be forwarded to the facility in advance.

CHAPTER 6

General Office Policies and Procedures

OVERVIEW

Helping to keep the office running smoothly is an important part of the medical administrative assistant's job. Tasks include opening the office; checking messages from the phone, email, and fax; and cleaning up the reception area. Once the patients start arriving, they must be greeted and assisted. Throughout the day, there are phone calls to answer, letters to write, and paperwork to complete.

This chapter explains many of these tasks, giving you a good idea of what a typical day looks like. After reading this chapter, you will understand many aspects of the medical administrative assistant's job.

By the end of this chapter, you should be able to answer the following questions.

1. What are three tasks that have to be done before closing the office for the day?
2. True or False: The accounting system does not have to be addressed until the end of the day.
3. Why is the telephone important to the medical office?
4. What components are included in a business letter?
5. Why do medical administrative assistants need to know how to use a word processing program?
6. True or False: Sending a fax is the most secure way to exchange information.
7. What are three acceptable times that information can be shared, as set forth by HIPAA?
8. What is the primary use for spreadsheets?
9. According to HIPAA, what information is a provider *not* allowed to share without the patient's permission?
10. Why would a medical practice use social media?

OPENING AND CLOSING PROCEDURES

Starting the Day

Most offices are locked at night, so the first task for the medical administrative assistant is to unlock the office and turn off the alarm, if the office has one. First and foremost, employees must prepare for patients and visitors.

Early-morning jobs include the following.

- Check the voicemail or answering service for any messages. Sometimes an answering service sends messages by email or fax. As you listen to each message, make sure you record the name of the person who called, the time and date of the call, and what the caller wanted on a phone message book.

- Make sure the phone has been redirected to the office from the answering service. During the workday, all phone calls should come in to the office.

- Print two copies of the day's appointments and place one on the provider's desk. Alternatively, you can have the appointment page of an electronic calendar ready for viewing. Use the second copy to pull medical records for patients who have appointments. If electronic medical records are used, make sure the provider knows how to access them. For paper records, make sure there is enough room in the progress notes sections for the provider to record what happens during the visit. If necessary, add an extra sheet for notes.

- Make sure that the front office is free of any obstacles that could impede or trip patients or employees.

- Check the restrooms to make sure they are stocked with toilet paper, soap, and hand towels.

- Clean the reception area so that it looks tidy when the first patient arrives. This involves straightening the magazines and making sure the sign-in sheets are in place. Sometimes the provider's business cards are put out for patients and visitors. Make sure there are enough cards for the day.

- Double-check that prescription pads are out of sight and reach of patients. Providers using electronic health records can print prescriptions directly from the computer system.

- Turn on necessary equipment, such as computers, laboratory equipment, and copy machines. Lights should be turned on in all the examination rooms.

- When turning on the computer, make sure a backup system for files is in place.

- Prepare the patient accounting system for the day. This includes balancing the day sheets, securing enough encounter forms for each patient with an appointment, and ensuring that the amount of petty cash available is correct.

Keeping Track of Supplies

One person should be responsible for ordering supplies, and an inventory should be kept so that supplies can be ordered as they run out. One way to do this is to record all the supplies the office uses onto a spreadsheet. The spreadsheet should include the name of the item, the number of items in stock, the usual price per item, and any bulk discounts.

Then follow these steps to determine when and how to order supplies.

1. Decide the point at which the supply should be replenished. Highlight those items to let office staff know.

2. Review the spreadsheet to determine which items should be reordered. When the order has been placed, note the date and quantity in the appropriate column on the spreadsheet.

3. When the order is received, note the date and quantity in the appropriate column. If the order is only partially filled, make note of the items that are back-ordered. Keep track of the order until it arrives.

4. Repeat the inventory and ordering process each month. Periodically, ask staff members for suggestions about specific supplies that should be ordered for the facility.

To purchase supplies, most providers establish accounts with suppliers. If possible, the balance should be paid off each month.

Closing the Office

At the end of the day, several tasks must be completed before locking up for the night. These include the following.

- Check to make sure that all patients have left the facility. Walk through all exam rooms and treatment areas to make sure they are empty.
- Turn off office equipment and take care of any other housekeeping chores that need to be done.
- Lock the file cabinets that contain patient records.
- Run account reports and balance the day sheet.
- Get ready for any bank deposits that need to be made.
- Turn the phones over to the answering service or to voicemail.

What are two tasks that need to be done to get the office ready for the day?

ANSWER: The phone, email, and fax messages need to be checked. Also, patient exam rooms need to be stocked with supplies the provider will need throughout the day.

GREETING PATIENTS

Courteous Behavior to All Patients

It is very important that every patient be treated courteously. Each patient should receive a friendly greeting, and by name if you know the patient. In most instances, it's best to use the patient's last name and title, such as "Ms. Jones" or "Mr. Vasquez."

It's a good idea to have a staff member at the reception desk at all times. Make sure the front desk is open so that arriving patients can see the receptionist. In turn, the receptionist should say hello to the patient, find out whether the visit is for an illness or a checkup, and have the patient sign in. Also, it's important to ask whether the patient is new or has been to the office before. If the patient is established, his or her chart can be pulled. If the patient is new, she might need to fill out paperwork or give the receptionist forms that have already been filled out.

Wait Times

Patients don't like to be kept waiting, though sometimes it's unavoidable. Do your best to bring the patient to the exam room for treatment or consultation as close to the appointment time as possible. If there will be a delay, let the patient know and keep him informed about long the delay will be. Any delay longer than 15 minutes should be explained. This acknowledges that you recognize that the patient's time is valuable.

Long waits can be more than simply annoying. They can cause patients undue fear and anxiety. Therefore, it is important to schedule patients as efficiently as possible, and do everything possible to put patients at ease. See Chapter 1 for more information about scheduling.

Why is it important to inform patients about wait times?

ANSWER: If a patient has to wait more than 15 minutes, the courteous thing to do is to let the patient know. This acknowledges that you recognize that the patient's time is valuable. Waiting a long time can also cause undue fear and anxiety. Therefore, it is important to do everything possible to put the patient at ease.

TELEPHONE ETIQUETTE

The telephone is the main communication device for most medical practices. Most patients make their appointments over the telephone. Therefore, it is essential that the medical administrative assistant be warm and welcoming when speaking to patients. When used appropriately, the phone can help build the medical practice. When used inappropriately, it can drive patients away. Telephone calls must be considered a key part of your workday. Never view them an interruption or an annoyance. If you do, that will be conveyed to the patient.

Most calls come from the following sources.

- Established patients calling for appointments or to ask questions

- New patients making a first contact with the provider's office

- Patients and medical workers reporting treatment results or emergencies

- Other providers making referrals or discussing a patient

- Laboratories reporting vital patient information

When answering the phone, be sure to speak in a pleasant, friendly voice. Speak clearly, pronouncing each word separately and distinctly. Do not speak in a monotone voice. Use *inflection*, or a change in pitch and loudness, as a way to emphasize certain points during the conversation. Avoid jargon, talk slowly and naturally, and avoid phrases such as "uh-huh" and "you know."

inflection. Use and change of tone or pitch in the voice.

jargon. Specific words or expressions used by a particular profession or group and that can be difficult for others to understand.

It is also important to be tactful when on the phone with a patient. That individual might be worried or agitated. Part of the medical administrative assistant's job is to attend to the patient's needs and make them feel comfortable. If you are busy when the phone rings, take a few seconds before answering the phone. Then you'll be able to answer graciously, without seeming breathless or impatient.

Identify the Facility

After picking up the phone, the first thing you should do is identify the facility, followed by your name. Numerous greetings can be used. Some providers prefer a formal greeting, while others allow a more causal opening.

Here are examples of typical telephone greetings.

- "This is Dr. Simon's office, Miss Myers speaking. How may I help you?"

- "Simon Maternal Health Clinic, this is Sarah Myers. How may I help you?"

- "Karen Simon's office, this is Miss Myers. How may I help you?"

- "Dr. Simon's office, this is Sarah. How may I help you?"

Some providers don't want their staff to use "Dr." in their greetings. This is a way to protect the patient's privacy, in case the call is going to an office where calls aren't always private. But it is still important to identify the facility so the patient knows that the call is from a medical provider.

Identify the Caller and the Reason for the Call

If a caller doesn't identify herself, ask who is calling. Ask the person whether she is a new patient, an established patient, or a salesperson. Then write down the name on a phone message pad. Repeat the name during the conversation to make sure you got it right and to give the call a friendly tone.

Also, if the caller is a family member of the provider, a protocol will generally be in place to interrupt the provider to take the call immediately or as soon as he finishes with a patient. If the caller is another physician, the protocol may be to interrupt. In other practices, the provider may phone back at the end of the current appointment. Most patient and pharmacy calls are returned by a medical administrative assistant, nurse, or other staff member by the end of the day.

Occasionally, the caller might refuse to give her name. When that happens, make every effort to identify the individual and find out the reason for the call. If the caller still refuses to identify herself, suggest sending a letter to the provider marked "personal." This request usually results in the person giving a name.

Next, find out the reason for the call. If it is a patient who would like to talk to the provider, find out if the provider is available to talk. If not, politely ask the patient to leave a message. Try to get a sense of when would be a good time for the provider to return the call.

If the call needs to be transferred to another staff member, give that individual a brief reason for the call before transferring it. When the conversation is over, be sure to end it in a pleasant manner.

Minimizing Time "On Hold"

If a caller chooses to wait on the line instead of waiting for a callback, make sure the person doesn't wait too long. Don't let more than 1 minute go by without checking in with the caller to give her an update on the status of the call. If the wait is longer than expected, the caller may decide to leave a message after all. If you take a message, make sure to get all the relevant information, which includes the following.

- Name of the person to whom the call is directed
- Name of the person calling
- Caller's daytime, evening, and/or cell phone number
- Reason for the call
- Date and time of the call
- Initials of the person taking the call

Another option is to transfer the call to another staff member who might be able to help the caller. For example, if the caller has a billing question, you may want to transfer the call to the person who handles those issues.

Why is it important to have good phone etiquette?

ANSWER: Most patients—both new and established—contact the office by phone. The person who answers the phone creates the first impression of the office. If that person is polite and courteous, patients are more likely to call back and return to the medical practice. But if the person who answers the phone is not polite, it will have the opposite effect, potentially leading to the loss of patients.

CREATING CORRESPONDENCE

Written communication also reflects on the medical practice. All letters, memorandums, replies to inquiries, responses to requests for information, telephone messages, emails, transcriptions, orders for supplies, and instructions to patients should be written carefully and concisely. Correspondence should be concise but not curt, with all the relevant information presented clearly.

In today's offices, most correspondence is written at the computer. Microsoft Word is the most common word-processing software. It is important to know how to use this software to compose letters.

Some offices have a standard form, or a *template*, that can be used as a model for letters. These are usually stored in a Word file labeled "templates." When you need to write a letter or other form of correspondence, go to this file and find the template you need. Then rename it and proceed with your work.

> *template.* A document with a preset format that is used as a starting point so that it does not have to be recreated each time.

Writing a Business Letter

A business letter may be written for many different purposes. Sometimes you may need to follow up with an insurance company about a claim. Other times, you may be answering questions from a supplier. For all professional correspondence, follow these steps.

1. Determine the purpose of the correspondence. Do so by looking at any letters that need to be answered. Highlight any questions that need to be addressed.

2. Make any notes on the letter you're responding to, or on a copy of it. You may also need a piece of scrap paper.

3. Prepare a draft of the letter using your desired letter format. Full block, in which all letter parts begin at the left margin, is generally preferred for professional correspondence. Other formats include simplified and modified block with indented or blocked paragraphs. A business letter usually has the following parts.

   a. The *heading* includes the letterhead and the dateline. The printed letterhead is usually centered at the top of the page. It includes the name or the provider or group and the address. It can include the telephone number and the medical specialty or specialties. In a group or corporate practice, the names of the providers may be listed. Occasionally, the heading includes the name of the office manager.

   b. The *opening* consists of the inside address and the salutation. The inside address includes the name of the individual or firm to whom the letter is addressed and the mailing address. When the letter is addressed to an individual, the name should be preceded by a courtesy title, such as Dr., Mr., or Ms. When addressing a letter to a provider, omit the courtesy title and type the provider's name, followed by his or her academic degree, such as MD or PhD. An example is Mark E. Jones, MD. Do *not* write, Dr. Mark E. Jones, MD. The salutation is the introductory greeting to the person being addressed. It is followed by a comma. An example of a salutation is "Dear Dr. Jones," or simply "Dr. Jones."

   c. The *body* of the letter describes the reason for the communication. Sometimes a subject line, such as "Re: Insurance Claim," may be used at the beginning of the letter. This alerts the reader to the purpose of the letter. Following the subject line, write a brief note explaining what you need to know.

    d. The *closing* includes the complimentary closing, typed signature, reference initials, and any special notations. The *complimentary closing* is the writer's way of saying goodbye. If you are on a first-name basis with the recipient of the letter, typical closings include "Cordially," "Very truly yours," or "Sincerely yours." If the letter is more formal, "Sincerely" is typically used.

    e. A *typed signature* is a courtesy to the reader, especially if the name does not appear on the printed letterhead of if the signature is hard to read.

    f. *Reference initials* of the writer and typist are placed below the typed signature.

    g. *Special notations* indicate that enclosures are included with the letter or that copies should be distributed to others. An enclosure is indicated by the word "Enclosure" or "enc," written below the reference initials. The copy notation is usually written as "cc:" or "copy to."

4. Make sure you've used good grammar and spelled everything correctly. Name and save the file.

5. Proofread a printed copy of the letter. Use proofreaders' marks to make corrections.

6. Make any necessary corrections. Then print it out and allow the provider or other relevant staff members to proofread it as well.

7. Make any final changes. Then print the letter on stationery.

8. Depending on the nature of the letter, either the provider or the medical administrative assistant will sign it. The provider signs the following kinds of letters.

    a. Those dealing with medical advice to patients

    b. Those to officers or committees of medical societies

    c. Referral and consultant reports to colleagues

    d. Medical reports to insurance companies

    e. Personal letters

> *complimentary closing.*
> The part of a letter that immediately precedes the signature, such as "Very truly yours," or "Sincerely."

Medical administrative assistants usually compose and sign letters about the following.

- Routine matters (e.g., arranging or rescheduling appointments)

- Orders for office supplies

- Notifications to patients about surgery or hospital arrangements

- Collection of delinquent accounts

- Letters of solicitation

FIGURE 6.1 *Business letter*

Jennifer McCain
490 West Ave.
Boston, MA 55555

February 3, 20XX

Dear Ms. McCain,

I am pleased to tell you that your enclosed Pap smear results are negative. Your next screening should be in about 1 year from today. Please contact our office if you have any questions or concerns.

Yours sincerely,

Amanda B Smith
Amanda B Smith, NP
cc Dr Horton

Enc.

Other Types of Communication

Letters aren't the only type of correspondence medical administrative assistants must compose. There are many other kinds.

Telephone messages

When taking telephone messages, they should always include the following pieces of information.

- Name of the person to whom the call is directed
- Name of the person calling
- Caller's daytime, evening, and/or cell phone number
- Reason for the call
- Date and time of the call
- Initials of the person taking the call

Email Messages

Emails are a popular form of communication. In a medical office, there are several advantages. First, they can be saved, printed for the patient's chart, and archived (saved over the long term) for storage. Emails that are pertinent to a patient's care or show a pattern of missed or canceled appointments should be printed and tracked.

Emails used for business should be written in the same formal style as business letters. Sometimes, however, it may be best to write a traditional letter because you have more control over confidentiality. It can be difficult to ensure that emails will be secure. If the email contains private information, include a disclaimer stating that it is confidential.

While you're at work, it's a good idea not to send personal emails. If you must send a personal email, be sure to use a separate account. Emails sent or received on a business account can be tracked, so a good rule to follow is don't engage in any communication that you don't want your employers to see. Some employers require employees to sign a statement that explains acceptable use of email and Internet. Employees may be terminated for not following rules about proper use of the computer system.

Faxed Messages

All faxes should have a cover sheet stating that the information in the fax is confidential and intended only for the person to whom it is sent. As with all communications, make sure it is well written and grammatically correct. Use fax only when absolutely necessary or when the information sent will not breach patient confidentiality. When sending faxes, a disclosure statement should be used. It also helps to call ahead when faxing information to alert the person who is to receive the fax. This practice helps ensure that the fax goes to the right person, which also promotes confidentiality.

Memorandums

Most offices send paper or electronic memorandums throughout the business week discussing when the office will be closed, when supplies will be ordered, and other information pertinent to the office. These forms of communication should be written clearly, concisely, and professionally. They should never convey a condescending attitude.

Applying Proper Postage

Most standard-sized envelopes require a first-class stamp. Forever stamps can be used even if the price of stamps goes up. If you're afraid that the letter might require additional postage, weigh it to make sure.

Using a roll of stamps, it is possible to stamp several envelopes at the same time. Tear off about 10 stamps, and fanfold the stamps on the perforations so that they separate easily. Fan the envelopes address-side up. Starting at one end of the fanned envelopes, attach the stamp at the end of the strip, tear it off, and proceed to the next envelope. Automated sealers and stampers are also available to make this procedure easier.

What are three types of communication you may be asked to write?

ANSWER: Three types of communication you may be asked to write are letters, emails, and memorandums.

BASIC COMPUTER SKILLS

Medical offices require workers to have a minimum level of computer skills. During the day, it is likely that you will be asked to write an email, send a memo, or look up something on the Internet.

Many offices use Microsoft Office. This software package includes an email system, word processing, and a program that can be used to develop spreadsheets. Each of these functions is described below.

Email system. Microsoft Outlook can sort email by date, subject, to whom you wrote, and from whom you received messages, and order of importance. Documents can be attached to encrypted emails and sent to patients, providers, and suppliers. Outlook also has a calendar function that can help you stay organized throughout the day. This can be used to track staff meetings, times when the provider is out of the office, times when other staff members are on vacation, and days when the office is closed.

Word processing. Microsoft Word allows you to create documents and do some formatting. For example, you can create different-colored heads and the "Insert" function to add tables and charts. It's important to be familiar with Word for writing letters and memos, as well as reports and progress notes the provider might need. After creating a document, be sure to name it and store it in the appropriate electronic folder. It will be identified as a document because it will have the extension .doc or .docx after it. Staying organized electronically and on paper is key to finding what you need quickly.

Spreadsheets. Microsoft Excel is a series of spreadsheets, which can be used to store patients' health information. Reports from laboratories or medical centers can be entered into a patient spreadsheet. When making such entries, it is essential that it be done carefully and accurately. In addition, all data must be entered as it is made available. Because confidentiality is such a big issue when dealing with patient information, some practices take extra precautions to ensure that information remains private. *Firewalls*, which are similar to filters, only allow certain types of data to enter or exit. Information can be *encrypted*, which means that it is changed into a code that can only be read after it is unencrypted. These precautions help protect this very sensitive information.

encrypted. Electronic data that has been encoded such that only authorized parties can read it

Use of the Internet

The Internet is another tool that is used in a medical office. For medical administrative assistants responsible for ordering supplies, the Internet can be used to shop for the best prices. Medical administrative assistants also may be asked to conduct research on the Internet. By entering a word or phrase into a search engine, various Web sites containing that word or phrase will appear on the results screen.

If you're conducting research, it's important to know which websites are reliable. Information from sites such as the American Heart Association and the American Medical Association are reliable, as are government websites, such as the National Institutes of Health (NIH) and the Centers for Disease Control and Prevention (CDC).

Some medical practices have websites, Facebook, or LinkedIn accounts as ways to advertise their business. Social media can be used to make announcements, such as when the office is closed or when a provider will be away. But because so much of providers' information concerns patients, they must be careful to follow security procedures and to follow the Health Insurance Portability and Accountability Act (HIPAA) regulations. These are explained in more detail in the next section.

HIPAA Regulations and Electronic Information

The purpose of HIPAA regulations is to protect patient information. For this reason, there are regulations in place regarding health information. It can be used and shared for the following reasons.

- For patient care and treatment coordination

- To pay providers and facilities for health care

- Among family, friends, and relatives whom the patient has identified as being involved in his health care

- To make sure good care is provided in clean facilities

- To protect public health

- To make required reports to law enforcement officials

In most cases, providers cannot share information without patients' permission. Specifically, the provider cannot:

- Give information to a patient's employer.

- Use or share health information for marketing purposes.

- Share mental health information obtained in counseling sessions.

Providers must be sure to train staff who use the computer about what information can and cannot be shared. Individual computer users should have their own login names and passwords that are not given to anyone else. All staff members should be required to use their login name and password every time they use the computer system. In addition, patient information must not be accessed unless the user needs something specific from a patient's file.

Be careful when releasing information. Only the minimum necessary information to accomplish a task may be accessed at any time. Audit trails are mandated in all software programs and track who accessed the information. It is illegal to access information about a person strictly because it is available. If any questions arise, direct them to the office manager or provider.

Use of Hardware

Most offices use equipment throughout the course of the workday. These include copiers, fax machines, printers, and scanners. Medical administrative assistants need to have a basic working knowledge of each of these.

Copiers are used to print multiple copies of documents. Copiers must be maintained so that the copies are always crisp and clear. This means that the toner cartridge must be replaced or refilled when necessary.

Fax machines allow people to exchange data through telephone lines. When sending a fax, it is important to take as many precautions as possible. This involves verifying the correct numbers, directing the fax to a certain person, and using cover sheets that stress confidentiality. Fax machines should be located in secure areas to prevent unauthorized access to health information.

Scanners can capture images of written text and photos at high resolution. They are often used to create electronic copies images so that older paper documents can be stored. Documents created from information captured by scanners can then be sent out by encrypted email.

Printers can print computer-generated files, or can be part of a fax, copy, and scanning device. Many all-in-one printers have photo-quality printing, print on both sides of the paper, and have wireless connectivity.

What computer programs does a medical administrative assistant need to know?

ANSWER: A medical administrative assistant must know how to use an email program such as Outlook, a word processing program such as Word, and a data entry program such as Excel.

SUMMARY

This chapter covered many of the basic tasks that a medical administrative assistant may be asked to perform during the workweek. These include preparing the office for the day and closing up at night; greeting patients appropriately and asking for relevant information; using proper etiquette when talking on the telephone; creating letters and other forms of correspondence; and using the computer system competently.

The next chapter covers basic medical terminology you will need to know to talk with patients, correspond with providers and insurance carriers, and read and type reports for the provider. This information will round out most of what you need to know to have a career as a medical administrative assistant.

CHAPTER DRILL QUESTIONS

Opening and Closing Procedures

1. What are three tasks that have to be done before closing the office for the day?

2. True or False: The accounting system does not have to be addressed until the end of the day.

Telephone Etiquette

3. Why is the telephone important to the medical office?

Creating Correspondence

4. What components are included in a business letter?

   a. Salutation and closing

   b. Body and closing

   c. Opening, salutation, body, complimentary closing, reference initials, and signature

   d. Salutation, body, and reference initials

Basic Computer Skills

5. Why do medical administrative assistants need to know how to use a word processing program?

6. True or False: Sending a fax is the most secure way to exchange information.

7. What are three acceptable times that information can be shared, as set forth by HIPAA?

8. What is the primary use for spreadsheets?

   a. Create typed reports and memos

   b. Send electronic messages

   c. Copy high-quality photos

   d. Enter and store data in table form

9. According to HIPAA, what information is a provider *not* allowed to share without the patient's permission?

10. Why would a medical practice use social media?

CHAPTER DRILL ANSWERS

1. Answer: Before leaving for the day, check to make sure that all patients have left the facility; straighten up the exam rooms so that they are ready for patients the next day; and lock the file cabinets that contain patient records.

2. Answer: False. The accounting system must be prepared for the day. This includes balancing the day sheets, securing enough encounter forms for each patient with an appointment, and ensuring that the amount of petty cash available is correct.

3. Answer: The telephone is the chief way patients communicate with the provider. Being polite and courteous can encourage patients to come back, while being rude can chase them away.

4. **A.** INCORRECT: This would be an incomplete business letter. The opening and body are missing, as well as the complimentary closing and signature.
   B. INCORRECT: This is incomplete. The salutation, complimentary closing, and signature are missing.
   C. CORRECT: This is all the elements of a business letter.
   D. INCORRECT: The opening, complimentary closing, and signature are missing from this list.

5. Answer: Medical administrative assistants need to know a word processing program because writing letters, memos, and reports is an important part of their job. All of these tasks typically are done on the computer.

6. Answer: False. Other people can read faxes, even if they are specifically sent to a certain person. Faxing should be done carefully and sparingly.

7. Answer: Information can be shared for patient care and treatment coordination; to pay providers and facilities for health care; and among family, friends, and relatives whom the patient has identified as being in involved in his or her health care.

8. **A.** INCORRECT: A word-processing program is used most often for this purpose.
   B. INCORRECT: An email program is used for this purpose.
   C. INCORRECT: A scanner is used to create photos.
   D. CORRECT: This is the most common use of spreadsheets.

9. Answer: Providers are not allowed to give information to a patient's employer; use or share health information for marketing purposes; and share mental health information obtained in counseling sessions.

10. Answer: A medical practice would use social media to advertise the practice and make announcements, such as when the office is closed or when specific providers are away.

CHAPTER 7
Basic Medical Terminology

OVERVIEW

Every profession has a specialized vocabulary, and medicine is no exception. Its language comes from ancient Greek or Latin terms. Hippocrates (460-377 BC), sometimes called "the father of medicine," was the first to standardize medical terminology. He also wrote the Hippocratic Oath, which providers pledge to follow. The Hippocratic Oath basically says that providers will do all they can to help patients, and above all, "will do no harm."

This chapter discusses the origins of medical terms. Often they are built by starting with a word root and then adding more specific prefixes and suffixes. For example, "cardio" is a word root meaning "heart." When the suffix "ologist," which means "one who studies," is added to cardio, the word "cardiologist" is formed. A cardiologist is a doctor who studies the heart.

Throughout this chapter, you will be learning more about common roots, prefixes, and suffixes. The chapter also goes over how to spell and pronounce common medical terms, and how to recognize and use abbreviations and acronyms. Knowledge of these words will help in communicating with both patients and providers.

By the end of this chapter, you should be able to answer the following questions.

1. What are two methods of learning proper terminology pronunciation?
2. True or False: Adding an -s to a word is the only way to make a medical term plural.
3. What two word parts are combined to build medical terms?
4. What does the abbreviation BP mean?
5. Why is it important for medical administrative assistants to understand abbreviations?
6. What does SOAP stand for?
7. What is PHI?
8. What does a neurologist do?
9. If the root "radio" means x-ray, what does the term *radiograph* mean?
10. If the root "path/o" means disease, what does the word *pathology* mean?

Hippocratic Oath. Providers promise to do all they can to help patients and "do no harm."

USING MEDICAL TERMINOLOGY WITH PATIENTS AND PROVIDERS

In a medical setting, saying and spelling words correctly is more than just a nice thing to do. In some cases, it can be a matter of life or death. Patients need to receive accurate information about their diagnosis and treatment plan. Providers must be confident that written documentation is correct.

For these reasons, pronunciation and spelling must always be accurate. In the next sections, strategies are given for how to master both of these skills.

Tips for Pronunciation

Practice is the best way to learn how to pronounce words correctly. Saying a word out loud each time you see it is a good way to become familiar with how the word sounds. There are some disagreements about pronunciation, as well as regional differences. If you're unsure how to pronounce something, ask a colleague. Also, make sure to keep a medical dictionary for help with pronunciation.

Dictionaries and other texts write out words phonetically to help with pronunciation. For example, the word *femoral* would be spelled FEM-or-al to indicate that the accent is on the first syllable. Diacritical marks to vowels are then added to help with their pronunciation. Vowels can be short, as in the words *cat* and *bar*, or long, as in *pace* or *plate*.

For the remaining vowels, here are some examples of words with long and short sounds.

- Short ĕ: ever, pet
- Long ē: equal, beet
- Short ĭ: kitten, pit
- Long ī: line, bite
- Short ŏ: pot, hot
- Long ō: boat, rose
- Short ŭ: cut, put
- Long ū: cute, cube

Tips for Spelling

As with pronunciation, the way to learn how to spell medical terms is by becoming familiar with them. Seeing them written down frequently is one way, as is writing them down. Checking spelling in a medical dictionary is always a good idea.

Understanding where terms come from is another way to remember how to spell them. Some medical terms are *eponyms*, or terms formed from names. Parkinson's disease is an example of an eponym.

Making Terms Plural

Most English words are made plural by adding an "s" or an "es." Some medical terms follow this rule, but others have different rules. Table 7.1 lists some rules for making medical terms plural.

TABLE 7.1 *How to make medical terms plural*

RULES FOR MAKING WORDS PLURAL	SINGULAR WORDS	PLURAL WORDS
Add -s to words ending in any vowel or consonant except -s, -x, -y, or -z.	Joint, face, angioma, cancer, muscle, paraplegic	Joints, faces, angiomas, cancers, muscles, paraplegics
Add -es to words ending in -s, -x, or -z.	Abscess, reflex	Abscesses, reflexes
Remove the -y and add -ies to words ending in -y preceded by a consonant. When an ending -y is preceded by a vowel, the usual plural suffix is -s.	Vasectomy, kidney	Vasectomies, kidneys
Remove the -x and add -ces to Latin words ending in -x.	Appendix, radix	Appendices, radices
Add -e to Latin terms ending in -a.	Fossa	Fossae
Remove -us and add -i to Latin words ending in -us.	*Staphylococcus*	*Staphylococci*
Remove -on and add -a to Greek words ending in –on.	Ganglion	Ganglia
Remove -um and add -a to Latin words ending in -um.	Datum	Data
Change -sis to -ses in Greek words ending in -sis.	Neurosis	Neuroses

Source: Medical terminology: A programmed approach, p. 6.

How would you make the word "cervix" plural?

ANSWER: Cervix would be made plural by dropping the -x and adding -ces. The word then becomes *cervices*.

eponym. Term formed from a name.

Identifying Medical Terms

Many medical terms are formed by building a word from a root and then adding a prefix to the beginning of the root and a suffix to the end. Often, a combining vowel links the root to the suffix.

Below are a few examples of how to build medical terms from these parts. More examples will be given later in the chapter.

A root contains the word's basic meaning. Here are some examples of roots.

- *Cardi* means heart.

- *Dent* means tooth.

- *Gastr* means stomach.

- *Laryng* means larynx.

- *Rhin* means nose.

By adding a connecting vowel or a suffix (word parts attached to the end of the word) beginning with a vowel, these roots can be combined to create medical terms. For example:

- *cardi* + suffix "ology" = *cardiology*, which means study of the heart.

- *dent* + suffix "algia" = *dentalgia*, which means a toothache.

- *gastr* + connecting vowel "o" + suffix "enterologist" = *gastroenterologist*, or someone who studies the digestive system.

- *laryng* + connecting vowel "o" + suffix "plasty" = *laryngoplasty*, or repair of the larynx.

- *rhin* + connecting vowel "o" + suffix "plasty" = *rhinoplasty*, or repair of the nose.

By adding prefixes (word parts attached to the beginning of a word), it is possible to create other medical terms. For example, in the word *disinfection,* the prefix "dis" means apart. When added to infection, the meaning becomes "removal of infection, or sterilization."

The prefix "retro" means behind. When put in front of a noun meaning a body part, such as peritoneum (the membrane that forms the lining of the abdominal cavity), the word becomes *retroperitoneum,* or the space behind the peritoneum

In addition to the suffixes mentioned earlier, there are many others. By adding the suffix "phobia," which means fear, to a word root, the meaning becomes the fear of something. For example, *acrophobia* means fear of heights and *claustrophobia* means fear of small spaces.

Prefixes before roots and connecting vowels and suffixes after roots can be combined to explain many different aspects of medicine. Here are some common ways they are used.

- To describe the structure and function of the body

- To describe body parts associated with a body system

- To describe system parts in detail

- To identify diagnostic, procedural, and laboratory terms

- To describe pathological terms

- To describe surgical terms

- To describe pharmacological terms

Later in this chapter, different roots, prefixes, and suffixes will be described, illustrating even more words that come together in this way.

What does the word cardiologist mean?

ANSWER: A cardiologist is someone who studies the heart.

ABBREVIATIONS AND ACRONYMS

Abbreviations and acronyms are both important forms of medical communication. Some abbreviations have become so common that the full name is almost never used. Similarly, in some cases, acronyms of organizations and terms have also taken the place of the complete name.

Abbreviations

Although abbreviations are widespread, they also have been associated with medical errors. As a result, several organizations have come out with recommendations about their use.

The abbreviations shown in Table 7.2 are used quite frequently, especially for prescription writing and patient instructions. But to avoid medical errors, abbreviations are now used less frequently in patients' medical records.

TABLE 7.2 *Common abbreviations*

ABBREV.	MEANING	ABBREV.	MEANING
a	before	Hx	history
ac	before meals	IM	intramuscular
AMI	acute myocardial infarction	LAC	laceration
bid	twice a day	LOC	level of consciousness
BP	blood pressure	mcg	micrograms
c/o	complaining of	NKDA	no known drug allergies
Ca	cancer/carcinoma	NPO	nothing by mouth
CC	chief complaint	po	by mouth
CHF	congestive heart failure	PRN	as needed
COPD	chronic obstructive pulmonary disease (emphysema, chronic bronchitis)	PT	physical therapy
CXR	chest x-ray	q	every
DOB	date of birth	qd	Every day
Dx	diagnosis	qid	four times a day
ECG, EKG	electrocardiogram	Rx	prescription
Fx	fracture	Tx	treatment
GI	gastrointestinal	sig	label
HEENT	head, ears, eyes, nose, throat	SOB	shortness of breath
h/o	history of	tid	three times a day
H&P	history and physical examination	w/o or s	without
HTN	hypertension	WNL	within normal limits

Using Abbreviations Throughout the Day

There are several reasons why it's important for medical administrative assistants to be familiar with abbreviations. First, providers often use them in their notes and prescriptions. Medical administrative assistants need to understand what these terms mean if they need to put them into an electronic record or explain them to a pharmacist.

Second, medical administrative assistants may be asked to explain instructions to patients. If abbreviations are used, patients will probably ask medical administrative assistants to interpret them. Patients might be confused or concerned about these abbreviations, so medical administrative assistants have the important job of not only explaining them, but also putting patients at ease and eliminating some of their concerns.

What does c/o mean?

ANSWER: c/o stands for "complaining of."

What does tid stand for?

ANSWER: tid stands for "three times a day."

Standardized Medical Terminology

Systematized Nomenclature of Medicine Clinical Terms® (SNOMED) is a detailed medical terminology standard developed for use in electronic medical records. SNOMED is intended to be used internationally for all medical coding and electronic transfer of medical data.

By 2013, 78% of providers had adopted some level of EHR. The current standard used for diagnosis coding is the International Classification of Diseases (ICD).

Acronyms

Many different kinds of acronyms are used in the health care industry. Some refer to medical record-keeping approaches, and others refer to terms commonly used by insurance carriers. Still others are laws and government agencies that medical administrative assistants should know about.

The following lists, organized by these three topics, identify some acronyms that medical administrative assistants need to know to do their job.

Medical Record-Keeping Approaches

SOAP is an approach often used for progress notes. The "S" stands for *subjective* impressions. The "O" stands for *objective* clinical evidence. The "A" stands for *assessment* or diagnosis. The "P" stands for *plans* for further studies, treatment, or management.

Some offices add an "E" to this protocol, which stands for *evaluation* or *education*. This notation documents that the patient was educated about his or her condition and given a patient information sheet.

Sometimes, an "R" may be added for *response*. This section is used to document an assessment of the patient's understanding of and compliance with the treatment plan.

POMR stands for problem-oriented medical record. It divides the medical record into four sections.

- The *database* includes the chief complaint, present illness, patient profile, review of systems, physical examination, and laboratory reports.

- The *problem list* is a numbered, titled list of every problem the patient has that requires management or workup. This can include social and demographic troubles, as well as medical or surgical ones.

- The *treatment plan* includes management, additional workups needed, and therapy. Each plan is titled and numbered with respect to the problem.

- The *progress notes* include structured notes that are numbered to correspond with each problem number.

CHEDDAR is another organizational approach to keeping medical records.

- *C:* Chief complaint

- *H*: History

- *E*: Examination

- *D*: Details (of problem and complaints)

- *D*: Drugs and dosages

- *A*: Assessment

- *R*: Return visit information, if applicable

SOAP. An approach used for progress notes: subjective, objective, assessment, plans.

POMR. Problem-oriented medical record. It divides the medical record into four sections.

CHEDDAR. An organizational approach to keeping medical records: chief complaint, history, examination, details, drugs and dosages, assessment, return visit information.

PHI stands for protected health information, and it is the term used by the Health Insurance Portability and Accountability Act (HIPAA). The PHI is any information about health status, the provision of health care, or payment for health care that can be linked to an individual patient. The medical office legally obligated to keep this information private.

Insurance Information

When reviewing insurance claims or explaining insurance information to patients, the medical administrative assistant must be familiar with many acronyms used by the industry. The following list covers many of the common terms that you need to know.

Health Insurance Portability and Accountability Act (HIPAA). Passed in 1996, this legislation was designed to improve the portability and continuity of health insurance coverage. It also serves to protect against waste, fraud, and abuse in health insurance and health care delivery; to protect the privacy of patients; and to simplify the administration of health insurance.

Throughout the day, HIPAA guides the following activities that medical administrative assistants perform.

- *How sign-in is conducted:* As much as possible, HIPAA requires that the identity of each patient remains private. As a result, sign-in sheets, where the names can be peeled off, are often used.

- *Filing systems:* To protect privacy, files should be turned away from the halls so that names can't be read.

- *Phone conversations*: As much as possible, be discreet when talking on the phone to a patient or about a patient's care.

- *Electronic information:* The proper precautions must be taken to ensure that it is protected.

Health maintenance organization (HMO). An organization that provides a wide range of comprehensive health care services for a specified group. This group pays fixed, periodic payments to the HMO. The HMO can be sponsored by the government, medical schools, hospitals, employers, labor unions, consumer groups, insurance companies, and hospital-medical plans. Knowledge of the basics about HMOs that patients use for insurance is needed to process claims and communicate with the HMO.

Preferred provider organization (PPO). Under this model, the health insurance carrier brings together providers, who agree on a predetermined list of charges for all services, including those for both normal and complex procedures. Typically these plans have a deductible and a coinsurance, often a 80%-20% split between the provider and patient. Many patients have insurance based on this model, so it's important for medical administrative assistants to understand concepts such as when a referral or a preauthorization is needed and how to take into account deductibles and coinsurance when billing.

Government Agencies and Professional Organizations

Government agencies oversee many aspects of the U.S. health care system. Although medical administrative assistants might not need to contact these agencies directly, it is helpful to know which is responsible for different functions. In addition, some professional organizations have oversight over specific areas. This list identifies a few of the most important agencies and organizations.

American Medical Association (AMA). The AMA is the professional organization for the nation's medical providers. It is concerned with ensuring high-level treatment at affordable prices. The AMA also sets the standards for ethics for the profession. Finally, the AMA publishes the Current Procedural Terminology (CPT), the codes used for procedures and services. Medical administrative assistants need to be aware of the work the AMA, especially its work with CPT codes. Providers use these codes to identify procedures and services, which are then used by insurance carriers to determine payment. Medical administrative assistants should check the codes on any claims documents to ensure that the most up-to-date ones are being used.

Centers for Disease Control and Prevention (CDC). Part of the Department of Health and Human Services, the CDC is concerned about the health and safety of people worldwide. It is a clearinghouse of information and statistics about infectious diseases, such as sexually transmitted diseases (STDs), HIV, and tuberculosis. It is an important resource for communities about upcoming health concerns, such as flu outbreaks. Medical administrative assistants should be aware of the services the CDC provides and check in with the organization if they are any concerns about epidemics.

Department of Health and Human Services (HHS). The HHS is the main U.S. agency charged with the protecting the health of all Americans. They are involved in the following.

- Medical and social science research
- Immunization services
- Financial assistance for low-income families
- Child support enforcement services
- Improvement of infant and maternal health
- Child and elder abuse prevention services
- Assistance for elderly Americans

The HHS also oversees CMS. Medicare is the nation's largest health insurer. Medical administrative assistants are often called upon to process Medicare claims, including CMS-1500 form. Chapter 4 explains in more detail how to fill out this form and how to be in compliance with CMS regulations.

National Institutes of Health (NIH). Also an agency of the HHS, the NIH has as its mission to uncover new knowledge that will lead to better health for everyone. It has 27 institutes and centers, with thousands of research projects being conducted at the NIH's laboratories and clinics. The NIH also funds other research projects being conducted at universities, medical schools, and hospitals. Although medical administrative assistants may not have reason to work with the NIH in doing their day-to-day tasks, it's important to have a general idea of the work it does. The NIH is an invaluable resource to anyone in the medical profession.

What are two acronyms related to the insurance industry that you need to know?

ANSWER: HMO, or health maintenance organization, and PPO, or preferred provider organization, are two important acronyms related to the insurance industry.

USING WORD PARTS TO DEFINE MEDICAL TERMINOLOGY

Earlier in the chapter, we introduced word roots, as well as prefixes and suffixes. In this section, we will add new information that is useful to know.

The word root is the foundation for each medical term. When building medical terms, the process usually begins with the word root. Identifying the root can be very helpful when trying to figure out what a term means.

The combining vowel ties the word root to the associated prefix and suffix. Sometimes the vowel is part of the prefix and suffix, and sometimes it is added to provide the necessary link.

Many prefixes and suffixes are used with different word roots to create words with different meanings. For example, the suffix *ologist* means "one who studies or specializes in." As you'll see below, *ologist* can be added to many different roots, creating a range of new words.

Building Words

Let's look at some prefixes and how they can be added to word roots. Table 7.3 shows some common prefixes.

Combining Roots with Prefixes

Here are some word roots. Let's see how they can be combined with these prefixes.

- The root "natal" means birth. *Prenatal* means before birth. *Postnatal* means after birth.

- The root "dexter" means right. *Ambidextrous* means the ability to use both the right and left sides.

- The root "cardio" means heart. *Endocardial* means within the heart. *Pericardial* means around the heart.

- The root "glyco" means having to do with sugar. *Hypoglycemia* means not having enough sugar in the body.

TABLE 7.3 *Common prefixes*

PREFIX	MEANING
a, an	without
ambi	both, around
endo	within
exo	outside
hyper	above normal
hypo	below normal
peri	enclosing, around
pre	before
post	after

Combining Roots With Suffixes

You can also build words by adding suffixes to the end of roots. Table 7.4 shows some common suffixes.

Here are some ways the suffixes can be combined with roots.

- The root "vascul/o" means vessel, usually a blood vessel. *Vasculitis* means inflammation of blood vessels.

- The root "gastr/o" means stomach. The root "entero" means intestines. Put all the two roots together with the suffix "ology," and you get *gastroenterology*, the study of the digestive system.

- The root "nephr/o" means kidneys. *Nephrology* is the study of kidneys.

TABLE 7.4 *Common suffixes*

SUFFIX	MEANING
graph	recording instrument
ist	one who studies or specializes in
itis	inflammation
logy	study of
osis	condition, state, process
pathy	disease

- The root "hepat/o" means liver. *Hepatitis* is inflammation of the liver, a disease that can take many different forms.

- The root "neur/o" means nerve. *Neuropathy* is a disease of the nerves.

By knowing just a few roots, prefixes, and suffixes, you can build many words. As you become more experienced in the medical field, you'll come across many more roots, prefixes, and suffixes. These rules will serve you well as you build your medical vocabulary.

What does gastroenterology mean?

ANSWER: Gastroenterology means the study of the digestive system.

SUMMARY

This chapter has provided you with information on a set of tools related to language. It has discussed tips for spelling and pronunciation, as well as how to figure out what a term means by its root, prefix, and suffix. This information is helpful in learning medical terms and adding to your vocabulary.

The chapter also discussed common abbreviations and acronyms. Knowledge of these words is also important in drafting reports, filling out insurance claims, and talking with patients about their medical needs. With this information in hand, you are gaining the skills you need to excel in your profession.

CHAPTER DRILL QUESTIONS

Using Medical Terminology with Patients and Providers

1. What are two methods of learning proper terminology pronunciation?

2. True or False: Adding an -s to a word is the only way to make a medical term plural.

3. What two word parts are combined to build medical terms?

    a. Abbreviations and acronyms

    b. Prefixes and suffixes

    c. Prefixes and abbreviations

    d. Prefixes and roots, suffixes and roots, or both prefixes and suffixes with roots

Abbreviations and Acronyms

4. What does the abbreviation BP mean?

5. Why is it important for medical administrative assistants to understand abbreviations?

6. What does SOAP stand for?

7. What is PHI?

Using Word Parts to Define Medical Terminology

8. What does a neurologist do?

9. If the root "radio" means x-ray, what does the term *radiograph* mean?

10. If the root "path/o" means disease, what does the word *pathology* mean?

CHAPTER DRILL ANSWERS

1. Answer: Saying the word out loud and checking a medical dictionary to see how the word is spelled phonetically are two ways to learn how to spell a word correctly.

2. Answer: False. Adding an -es to words ending in -s, -x, or -y; removing the -y adding an -ies to words ending -y preceded by a consonant, and removing an -x and adding a -ces are three other ways to make medical terms plural.

3. **A.** INCORRECT: Abbreviations are shorthand for longer terms, and acronyms are abbreviations for organizations or procedures. They cannot be combined to build medical terms.
    B. INCORRECT: Prefixes go before roots and suffixes go after roots.
    C. INCORRECT: Combining prefixes with abbreviations would not result in any words.
    D. CORRECT: This is an accurate description of how medical terms are built.

4. Answer: BP stands for blood pressure.

5. Answer: First, providers often use abbreviations in their notes and prescriptions. Medical administrative assistants need to understand what these terms mean if they need to put them into an electronic record or explain them to a pharmacy. Second, medical administrative assistants may be asked to explain instructions to patients. If abbreviations are used, patients will probably ask medical administrative assistants to interpret them. Patients may be confused and concerned about these abbreviations, so medical administrative assistants have the important job of not only explaining them, but also putting patients at ease and eliminating some of their concerns.

6. Answer: This is an approach often used for progress notes. The "S" stands for subjective impressions. The "O" stands for objective clinical evidence. The "A" stands for assessment or diagnosis. The "P" stands for plans for further studies, treatment, or management.

7. Answer: This stands for protected health information, and it is the term used by the Health Insurance Portability and Accountability Act (HIPAA). The PHI is any information about health status, the provision of health care, or payment for health care that can be linked to an individual patient. The medical office legally obligated to keep this information private.

8. Answer: A neurologist is a doctor of the nervous system.

9. Answer: The suffix "graph" means recording instrument. Thus, the word radiograph means an instrument used to make an x-ray.

10. Answer: The suffix "ology" means study of. Thus, the word pathology means study of disease.

IN PRACTICE
Case Studies

CASE STUDY 1: SCHEDULING

Cindy, a CMAA, is working at an office that uses categorization booking. On Monday, Cindy enters two appointments into the electronic scheduling system for Friday. One patient needs a physical exam, and the other will receive a stress test. Cindy books the physical at 11 a.m. for 1 hr, and the stress test at 3 p.m. for 1 hr in the ultrasound room.

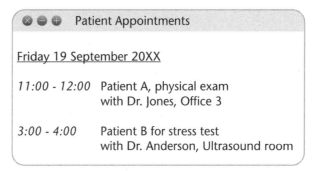

Two days pass. Jan, another CMAA, is preparing to book an ultrasound for the 3 p.m. time slot on Friday, and sees Cindy's booking error. When discussing the situation with Cindy, she tells her that Dr. Jones always takes his lunch break from 11 a.m. to noon. Therefore, the patient's physical at 11 a.m. will not work for Dr. Jones. Jan also explains that the room containing both ultrasound and stress testing equipment is reserved for ultrasound patients on Friday afternoons. Cindy understands and agrees to reschedule to two appointments she set.

To eliminate future scheduling errors, Jan suggests using a matrix grid in the online scheduling system to track when providers are unavailable. She also recommends adding a column for rooms that require major equipment.

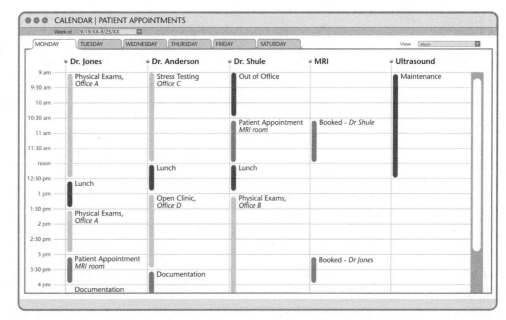

QUESTION 1 *What should the facility add to its online scheduling system to prevent future scheduling errors?*

A matrix grid with time slots designated by provider and room/equipment availability.

QUESTION 2 *When rescheduling the appointments, what should Cindy consider?*

Cindy should consider how her facility categorizes appointments. She also must consider the duration of each appointment she sets. She needs to give providers enough time in each room with the necessary equipment so that other commitments are not affected.

QUESTION 3 *What other scheduling options might Cindy consider?*

Cindy may choose to schedule the patient who wants a physical on another day or time when his provider is available. Or Cindy might have the patient see another provider if the patient isn't flexible on the day his provider is open. Cindy will need to advise the patient needing a stress test that those are only scheduled for Thursday mornings because there is only one room with equipment.

QUESTION 4 *Because the practice uses the categorization method of booking, what problems can arise by booking the ultrasound and stress test side-by-side at 3 p.m. on Friday?*

Booking the two separate types of appointments side-by-side can result in a double-booking model, and negates the decision to use categories. The other big drawback is the length of time it takes to perform the two services. The stress test takes much longer than the ultrasound and can result in longer waiting times.

CASE STUDY 2: CORRECT REFERRAL FORM

A patient, Shirley Levine, logs into her online patient portal to view her encounter form 10 days after her initial visit. Shirley's provider referred her to a gastroenterologist.

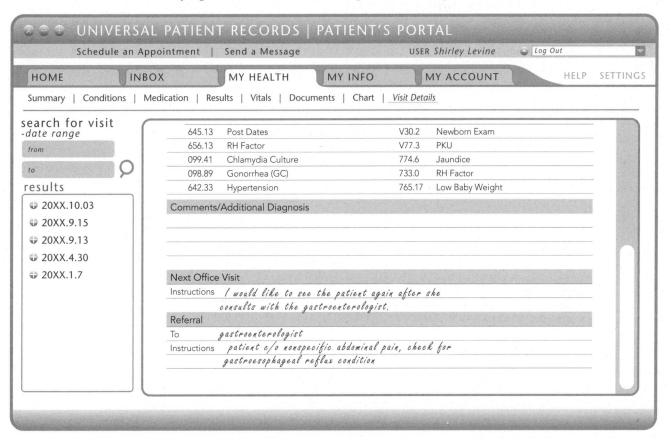

She gave this referral to the CMAA upon exiting the clinic. Shirley told the CMAA that she would await notification as to whether her services were covered before making an appointment with the specialist.

When the patient calls the CMAA to inquire, the CMAA discovers that she forgot to process the referral and contact the insurance carrier for authorization. This error delayed Shirley's services.

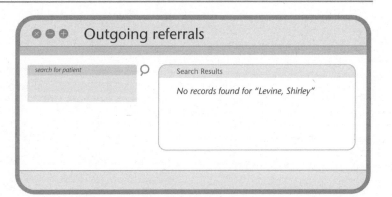

QUESTION 1 *What might have happened if Shirley made an appointment with the specialist before receiving preauthorization?*

The patient likely would have had to pay for some or all of her services. Insurance carriers are very clear that the burden of referral tracking is on the patient.

QUESTION 2 *What should the CMAA do to correct this error?*

The CMAA should immediately validate the patient's insurance over the phone and verify that the information in her record is correct. Next, she will want to process a referral over the phone.

QUESTION 3 *What kind of referral should the CMAA submit to the patient's insurance carrier after speaking with the patient?*

The CMAA should submit an urgent referral. She should explain her mistake to the insurance carrier, and hope the referral processing will be expedited.

QUESTION 4 *What information will the CMAA need to have available in order to process the referral?*

The CMAA will need to provide the patient's name, date of birth, Social Security number, insurance ID number, group ID number, diagnosis code related to the referral, provider referred to, referring provider, potential dates of service, and requested number of visits. The carrier may request chart notes or a discussion regarding particulars of the treatment to this point.

QUESTION 5 *How will the CMAA know if the patient's services are covered for this procedure?*

The insurance carrier will provide a verification or authorization number, and confirm specific procedures, services, and treatment sessions. The CMAA should document these on the referral form.

CASE STUDY 3: COMPLIANCE

Example 1

Janice, a Blue Cross Blue Shield representative, is missing information from Dr. Richardson's office. The office sent a nonspecific diagnosis about a gall bladder surgery. Janice calls Sarah, a CMAA, for clarification.

Diagnosis Clarification Claim #454565664 - Inbox

Health Insurance | Example Company
Sent: Mon, 29 Sep 20XX 20:17:02
To: Billing@HealthCareProviders.org
Subject: Diagnosis Clarification Claim #454565664

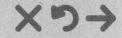

CONFIDENTIALITY NOTICE: This e-mail message including attachments, if any, is intended for the person or entity to which it is addressed and may contain confidential, privileged, and/or proprietary material. Any unauthorized review, use, disclosure or distribution is prohibited. If you are not the intended recipient, please contact the sender by reply e-mail and destroy all copies of the original message.

To Whom It May Concern:

We are in receipt of claim #454565664 for patient #SmiDa797 totaling $1257.92.

Further information is needed in order to process this claim.
 Invalid diagnosis code 789.00 - Abdominal pain, unspecified site.

Please provide the necessary information utilizing our automated claims unit available 24/7 for your convenience. Should you prefer to speak with a representative, you may call our provider services line between the hours of 8am and 5pm PST, Monday through Friday at 888-555-1234.

This claim will remain in development for 30 days. Failure to respond to this request may result in denial of payment.

Claims Department
Health Insurance | Example Company

Example 2

An oral surgeon wants to refer a patient to an orthodontist for braces. The surgeon asks Shondra, the CMAA, to fax the x-ray from the patient's report.

Example 3

A pharmacist completes a transaction with a patient, Mrs. Kim. After the patient leaves, the pharmacist notices the pharmacy's pseudoephedrine logbook open on the counter. The pharmacist asks the pharmacy technician, Eric, if he left the logbook out.

Oral Surgery Care Providers

1234 Main Street
Shermer, IL 12345
1.800.555.1234

Fax Cover Sheet

To	Name Phone Fax	Holt Orthodontics 321-555-1234 321-555-5678
From	Name Contact Phone Fax	Oral Surgery Care Providers Shondra Davis 456-555-0987 456-555-1234
	Patient Name Identifier Medical Record Number	Tara Mitchell 1234578 09876543
	Reason for Release	Referral

QUESTION 1 *Explain the HIPAA provision that allowed Sarah to easily respond to the requests of the insurance claims processor.*

Daily operations are the HIPAA provision of Treatment, Payment, and Operations (TPO). The law allows minimum necessary disclosure of PHI for these purposes, once the Notice of Privacy Practices has been signed, without further authorization.

QUESTION 2 *Explain how Dr. Banks's request to fax the x-ray report to Dr. Holt is allowable under HIPAA guidelines.*

Dr. Banks is making a referral to another provider. Faxing the x-ray report falls under the treatment provision of TPO.

QUESTION 3 *The fax Shondra is planning to send will contain PHI. Describe the steps she will need to take to be certain the transmitted PHI is secure.*

Shondra should call ahead to be certain someone is in the office to receive the fax. She will also need to verify the fax number is correct, and use a cover sheet that stresses confidentiality. Once the fax is transmitted, a best practice is to call and confirm receipt by the proper person.

QUESTION 4 *Describe the level of HIPAA violation Eric committed and the approximate penalty HHS might assess.*

While final penalties are determined on a case-by-case basis, HIPAA violations can be assessed to individuals and range from $100 to $1.5 million. Penalties can also include further monitoring and guidance on compliance deficiencies uncovered during an investigation.

QUESTION 5 *How might the pharmacy prevent future instances similar to Eric's violation?*

The violation of leaving the logbook with PHI exposed on the counter was carelessness. Perhaps the employees were not properly trained, or the store did not have policies and procedures in place to prevent this type of error. The store should evaluate these two areas and perform internal audits to identify other deficiencies.

APPENDIX
References

Aging With Dignity. Retrieved July 8, 2014, from http://www.agingwithdignity.org

AHIMA's long-term care health information practice & documentation guidelines. Retrieved July 11, 2014, from http://ahimaltcguidelines.pbworks.com/w/page/46493963/Record%20Systems%2C%20 Organization%20and%20Maintenance

American Health Information Management Association. (2011.) *Record Systems, organization and maintenance.* Retrieved July 29, 2014, from http://ahimaltcguidelines.pbworks.com/w/ page/46493963/Record%20Systems%2C%20Organization%20and%20Maintenance

Assurant Health. *Frequently asked health insurance questions.* Retrieved July 29, 2014, from http://www.assuranthealth.com/corp/ah/Customers/health-insurance-questions.htm

Booth, K. A., Whicker, L. G., Wyman, T. D., Pugh, D. J., Thompson, S. (2009.) Medical Assisting: Administrative and Clinical Procedures, 3rd Edition. *Chapter 12: Scheduling Appointments Powerpoint.* Slide 17. New York: McGraw-Hill Companies.

Bostwick, P., and Weber, H. (2013). *Medical terminology: A programmed approach.* 2nd Ed. New York: McGraw-Hill Companies, Inc.

Casto, A. B., and Forrestal, E. (2013.) *Principles of healthcare reimbursement.* (4th Ed.). pp. 75. Chicago, IL: AHIMA Press.

Centers for Medicare & Medicaid Services. (2013, November.) *Advance beneficiary notice of noncoverage (ABN).* Retrieved July 29, 2014, from http://www.cms.gov/Outreach-and-Education/ Medicare-Learning-Network-MLN/MLNProducts/downloads/abn_booklet_icn006266.pdf

Centers for Medicare & Medicaid Services. (April 2013). *ICD-10-CM/PCS: The next generation of coding.* Retrieved June 17, 2014, from https://www.cms.gov/Medicare/Coding/ICD10/downloads/ ICD-10Overview.pdf

Centers for Medicare & Medicaid Services. (Rev. 2013, Dec. 27.) *Medicare claims processing manual.* Chapter 26. Retrieved July 22, 2014, from http://www.cms.gov/Regulations-and-Guidance/ Guidance/Manuals/downloads/clm104c26.pdf

Equal Rights Center. (2011.) *Ill-prepared: Health care's barriers for people with disabilities.* Retrieved July 29, 2014, from http://www.equalrightscenter.org/site/DocServer/Ill_Prepared.pdf?docID=561

Geisinger Health Plan. *UB-04 claim form instructions.* Retrieved July 22, 2014, from https:// www.thehealthplan.com/documents/providers/ub04_instructions.pdf

Ill-Prepared: Health Care's Barriers for People with Disabilities. (2010.) Washington, D.C.: The Equal Rights Center. Retrieved July 8, 2014, from http://www.equalrightscenter.org/site/DocServer/ Ill_Prepared.pdf?docID=561

Insure.com. (August 3, 2012). *"Birthday rule" determines health insurance coverage.* Retrieved June 17, 2014, from http://www.insure.com/articles/healthinsurance/birthday-rule.html

Jobs Descriptions. (2008.) Retrieved June 17, 2014, from http://www.jobsdescriptions.org/assistant/ back-office-medical-assistant.html

Lindh, W., Pooler, M., Tamparo, C., Dahl, B., Morris. J. (2013.) *Delmar's comprehensive medical assisting: Administrative and clinical competencies.* Independence, KY: Cengage Learning.

Milum Corporation. (2012.) *Appointment scheduling with Office Tracker*. http://www.officetracker.com/html/appointmentscheduling.html

National Institutes of Health. *HIPAA Privacy Rule information for researchers*. Retrieved July 22, 2014, from http://privacyruleandresearch.nih.gov/pr_06.asp

PBworks. (2011.) Young-Adams, A. P. (2011.) *Kinn's The administrative medical assistant: An applied learning approach*. 7th Ed. St. Louis, MO: Elsevier/Saunders.

Reimbursement Concepts University. *The insurance verification process*. Retrieved June 17, 2014, from http://www.rcuonline.net/images/InsuranceVerificationProcess.pdf

Sanderson, S. M. (2012.) *Computers in the medical office*. (8th Ed.) New York: McGraw Hill.

Sayles, Nanette B. (Ed.) (2013). *Health information management technology: An applied approach* (4th ed.). Chicago: American Health Information Management Association.

Silver, L. (2013.) The Practice Solution Magazine. *Five steps to HIPAA Privacy Rule compliance*. http://magazine.thepracticesolution.net/2005/05/five-steps-to-hipaa-privacy-rule-compliance/

U.S. Department of Health & Human Services. *Health information privacy*. Retrieved July 22, 2014, from http://www.hhs.gov/ocr/hipaa/

Walls, A. (2014, Apr. 29.) *From hospitals to courtrooms, new tools to topple language barriers*. The Seattle Globalist. Retrieved July 29, 2014, from http://www.seattleglobalist.com/2014/04/29/new-tools-to-topple-language-barriers/23615

Young-Adams, A. P. (2011.) *Kinn's The administrative medical assistant: An applied learning approach*. 7th Ed. St. Louis, MO: Elsevier/Saunders.

APPENDIX
Glossary

A

abandonment. Discontinuing medical care without giving the proper notice or providing a competent replacement.

accounts receivable ledger. Document that provides detailed information about charges, payments, and remaining amounts owed to a provider.

active files. Section of medical charts for patients currently receiving treatment.

administrative services only (ASO) contract. Contract between employers and private insurers under which employers fund the plans themselves, and the private insurers administer the plans for the employers.

Advance Beneficiary Notice of Noncoverage (ABN). Form provided to a patient if a provider believes that a service may be declined because Medicare might consider it unnecessary.

advance directive form. Document that spells out what kind of treatment a patient wants in the event that he can't speak for himself. Also known as living will.

allowable amount. The limit that most insurance plans put on the amount that will be allowed for reimbursement for a service or procedure.

appointment cards. Used to remind patients of scheduled appointments and to eliminate misunderstandings about dates and times.

assault and battery. Willful and unlawful use of intimidation and physical force or violence on another person.

assets. The properties owned by a business.

assignment of benefits (AOB) form. Form that authorizes health insurance benefits to be sent directly to providers.

audit trail. A report that traces who has accessed electronic information.

B

benefit period. Time during which benefits are payable under a given insurance plan.

birthday rule. The health plan of the parent whose birthday comes first in the calendar year is designated as the primary plan.

Blue Cross and Blue Shield plan. The first prepaid plan in the U.S. that offers health insurance to individuals, small businesses, seniors, and large employer groups.

bookkeeping. Part of the office's accounting functions, to include recording, classifying, and summarizing financial transactions.

business associates. Individuals, groups, or organizations, who are not members of a covered entity's workforce, that perform functions or activities on behalf of or for a covered entity.

C

capitation. The fixed amount a provider receives.

certified mail. First-class mail that also gives the mail added protection by offering insurance, tracking, and return receipt options.

CHEDDAR. An organizational approach to keeping medical records: chief complaint, history, examination, details, drugs and dosages, assessment, return visit information.

closed files. Section of medical charts for patients who have died, moved away, or terminated their relationship with the physician.

cluster or categorization booking. Booking a number of patients who have specific needs together at the same time of day.

coinsurance. A form of cost-sharing that kicks in after the deductible has been met.

complimentary closing. The part of a letter that immediately precedes the signature, such as "Very truly yours," or "Sincerely."

consent. A patient's permission.

copayment. A fixed fee for a service or medication, usually collected at the time of service or purchase.

covered entities. Providers, hospitals, laboratories facilities, nursing homes, rehabilitation facilities, health plans, health care clearinghouses, and those that supply care, services, or supplies to a patient and transmit any health information electronically.

cross-reference. Reference to corresponding information in a separate location.

D

daily journal. A chronological record of bills received, bills paid, and payments and reimbursements received.

day sheet. A daily record of financial transactions and services rendered.

deductible. The amount a patient must pay before insurance pays anything.

differential diagnosis. The process of weighing the probability that other diseases are the cause of the problem.

direct filing system. System in which the only information needed for filing and retrieval is a patient's name.

disbursement. The record of the funds distributed to specific expense accounts.

divulge. Make private or sensitive information known.

DNR form. Form that states that the patient does not want to be revived after experiencing a heart episode or other kind of life-threatening event.

double-booking. Two patients are scheduled to come at the same time to see the same physician.

E

electronic data interchange (EDI). The transfer of electronic information in a standard format.

electronic health record (EHR). An electronic record of health-related information about a patient that conforms to nationally recognized interoperability standards that can be created, managed, and reviewed by authorized providers and staff from more than one health care organization.

electronic medical record (EMR). An electronic record of health information that is created, added to, managed, and reviewed by authorized providers and staff within a single health care organization.

emancipated minor. A person younger than the age of majority (usually 18 to 21 years of age) who is married, in the armed forces, living apart from parents or a guardian, or self-supporting.

employer-based insurance. Insurance that is tied to an individual's place of employment.

encounter form. A document used to collect data about elements of a patient visit that can become part of a patient record or be used for management purposes.

encrypted. Electronic data that has been encoded such that only authorized parties can read it

end-of-day summary. Document consisting of proof of posting sections, month-to-date accounts receivable proof, and year-to-date accounts receivable proof.

eponym. Term formed from a name.

equities. What is left of assets after creditors' liabilities have been subtracted.

explanation of benefits (EOB). A record of a patient's fees.

exposure control plan. Plan that describes tasks employees must perform if there is a risk of exposure to blood or other potentially infectious materials, and what procedures are in place to track employee exposures.

F

fee-for-service. Model in which providers set the fees for procedures and services.

firewall. Part of a computer system that blocks unauthorized access while allowing outward communication.

first-class mail. Sealed or unsealed typed or handwritten material, including letters, postal cards, postcards, and business reply mail.

fraud. Making false statements of representations of material facts to obtain some benefit or payment for which no entitlement would otherwise exist.

G

general journal. Document where transactions are entered.

guarantor. Person or entity responsible for the remaining payment of services after insurance has paid.

H

Healthcare Common Procedure Coding System (HCPCS). A group of codes and descriptors used to represent health care procedures, supplies, products, and services.

Health Care Fraud and Abuse Program (HCFAP). Program that protects Medicare and other HHS programs from fraud and abuse by conducting audits, investigations, and inspections.

Healthcare Integrity and Protection Data Bank (HIPDB). A compilation of information about fraud and abuse.

health history form. Form that asks patients to list any illnesses or surgeries they have had, family history, medications taken, chronic health issues, allergies, and other physicians they consulted.

health information exchange (HIE). System that enables the sharing of health-related information among providers according to nationally recognized standards.

Health Insurance Portability and Accountability Act (HIPAA) of 1996. Legislation that includes Title II, the first parameters designed to protect the privacy and security of patient information.

health maintenance organization (HMO). Plan that allows patients to only go to physicians, other health care professionals, or hospitals on a list of approved providers, except in an emergency.

HIPAA Security Rule. Rule that describes safeguards that must be in place to protect the confidentiality, integrity, and availability of health information stored in a computer and transmitted across computer networks, including the Internet.

Hippocratic Oath. Providers promise to do all they can to help patients and "do no harm."

I

implied consent. A patient presents for treatment, such as extending an arm to allow a venipuncture to be performed.

inactive files. Section of medical charts for patients the provider has not seen for 6 months or longer.

incidental disclosure. Secondary use of PHI that cannot be reasonably prevented, is limited in nature, and occurs as a result of another use or disclosure that is permitted.

individually identifiable health information. Documents or bits of information that identify the person or provide enough information so that the person could be identified.

inflection. Use and change of tone or pitch in the voice.

informed consent. Providers explain medical or diagnostic procedures, surgical interventions, and the benefits and risks involved, giving patients an opportunity to ask questions and consent before medical intervention is provided.

insured mail. Mail that has insurance coverage against loss or damage.

invoice. A document that describes items purchased or services rendered and shows the amount due.

J

jargon. Specific words or expressions used by a particular profession or group and that can be difficult for others to understand.

L

liabilities. The equity of those to whom money is owed (creditors).

living will. Document that spells out what kind of treatment a patient wants in the event that he can't speak for himself. Also known as advance directive.

M

managed care organization. Organization developed to manage the quality of health care and control costs.

matrix. A grid with time slots blocked out when physicians are unavailable or the office is closed.

Medicaid. A government-based health insurance option that pays for medical assistance for individuals who have low incomes and limited financial resources. Funded at the state and national level. Administered at the state level.

medical necessity. The documented need for a particular medical intervention.

Medicare Advantage (MA). Combined package of benefits under Medicare Parts A and B that may offer extra coverage for services such as vision, hearing, dental, health and wellness, or prescription drug coverage.

Medicare. Federally funded health insurance provided to people age 65 or older, people younger than 65 who have certain disabilities, and people of all ages with end-stage kidney disease.

Medicare Part A. Provides hospitalization insurance to eligible individuals.

Medicare Part B. Voluntary supplemental medical insurance to help pay for physicians' and other medical professionals' services, medical services, and medical-surgical supplies not covered by Medicare Part A.

Medicare Part D. A plan run by private insurance companies and other vendors approved by Medicare to cover the cost of approved prescriptions.

Medicare Summary Notice (MSN). Document that outlines all of the services and supplies, the amounts billed by the provider, the amounts paid by Medicare, and what the patient must pay the provider for the preceding 3-month period.

Medigap. A private health insurance that pays for most of the charges not covered by Parts A and B.

modified wave booking. Wave booking can be modified in a couple of different ways. One example of this approach is to schedule two patients to come at 9 a.m. and one patient at 9.30. This hourly cycle is repeated throughout the day.

modifiers. Added information or changed description of procedures and services, and are a part of valid CPT or HCPCS codes.

N

National Provider Identifier (NPI). Unique 10-digit code for providers required by HIPAA.

non-covered entities. Organizations that use, collect, access, and disclose individually identifiable health information, but do not transmit electronic data. These do not have to comply with the Privacy Rule.

Notice of Privacy Practices. Document informing a patient of when and how their PHI can be used.

O

Occupational Safety and Health Administration (OSHA). Part of the U.S. Department of Labor with the mission to ensure workplace safety and a healthy working environment.

open booking (tidal wave scheduling). Patients are not scheduled for a specific time, but told to come in at intermittent times. They are seen in the order in which they arrive.

out-of-pocket maximum. A predetermined amount after which the insurance company will pay 100% of the cost of medical services.

P

packing slip. A list of items in a package.

patient financial responsibility form. Form that confirms that the patient is responsible for payments to the provider.

Patient's Bill of Rights. A list of guarantees for people receiving medical care

perpetual transfer method. Identifying files for purging by marking the outside of the file.

petty cash fund. A small amount of cash available for expenses such as postage, parking fees, small contributions, emergency supplies, and miscellaneous small items.

POMR. Problem-oriented medical record. It divides the medical record into four sections.

preauthorization. Formal approval from the insurance company that it will cover the test or procedure.

preferred provider organization (PPO). Plan that allows patients to use physicians, specialists, and hospitals in the plan's network and receive a greater discount on services.

premium. A pre-established amount set by the insurance company and paid regularly, usually on a monthly basis, by the patient or an employer.

priority mail. First-class mail weighing more than 13 ounces.

Privacy Rule. A HIPAA rule that establishes protections for the privacy of individual's health information.

private fee-for-service plan. Plan that allows patients to go to any physician, other health care professional, or hospital as long as the providers agree to treat those patients.

private health insurance. Health insurance subsidized through premiums paid directly to the company.

program abuse. Practices that, either directly or indirectly, result in unnecessary costs to government-funded programs.

protected health information (PHI). Information about health status or health care that can be linked to a specific individual.

provisional diagnosis. A temporary or working diagnosis.

purging. The process of moving a file from active to inactive status.

R

registered mail. Mail of all classes protected by registering and requesting evidence of its delivery.

regular referral. When a physician decides that a patient needs to see a specialist.

reimbursement. Payment from insurance companies.

resource-based relative value scale (RBRVS). System that provides national uniform payments after adjustments across all practices throughout the country.

S

screening system. Procedures to prioritize the urgency of a call to determine when the patient should be seen.

shared decision-making. A patient and provider work together to decide on a treatment plan.

single-entry system. A method of bookkeeping that relies on a one-sided accounting entry to maintain financial information.

SOAP. An approach used for progress notes: subjective, objective, assessment, plans.

standard mail. Mail that includes advertising, promotional, directory, or editorial material, or any combination of such material.

State Children's Health Insurance Program (SCHIP). A program jointly funded by the federal government and the states to cover uninsured children in families with modest incomes too high to qualify for Medicaid.

statement. A request for payment.

stat referral. Needed in an emergency situation, and can be approved immediately over the telephone after the utilization review has approved the faxed document.

stream/time-specific scheduling. Scheduling patients for specific times at regular intervals. The amount of time allotted depends on the reason for the visit.

subsidiary journals. A document where transactions are summarized and later recorded in a general ledger.

T

template. A document with a preset format that is used as a starting point so that it does not have to be recreated each time.

U

unbundling. Using multiple codes that describe different components of a treatment instead of using a single code that describes all steps of the procedure.

upcoding. Assigning a diagnosis or procedure code at a higher level than the documentation supports, such as coding bronchitis as pneumonia.

urgent referral. When an urgent, but not life-threatening, situation occurs, requiring that the referral be taken care of quickly.

V

verbal consent. Consent for treatment given out loud in response to a pointed question.

W

wave booking. Patients are scheduled at the same time each hour to create short-term flexibility each hour.

APPENDIX
Index

Figures (f) and tables (t) are indicated following page numbers.

Certified Medical Administrative Assistant (CMAA) Study Guide